Prions - Some Physiological and Pathophysiological Aspects

Edited by Ivo Nikolaev Sirakov

Published in London, United Kingdom

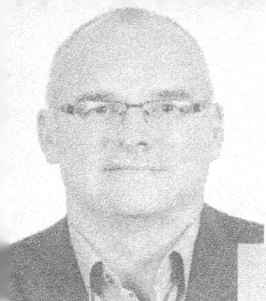
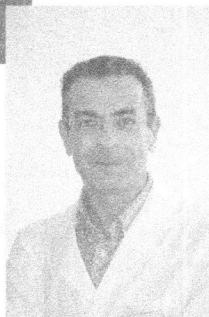
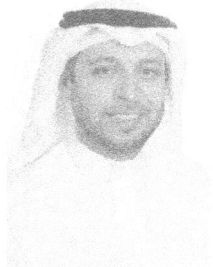
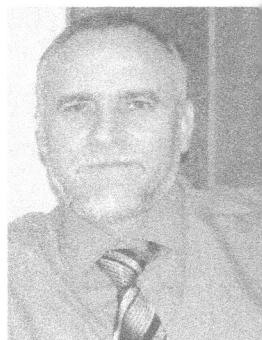
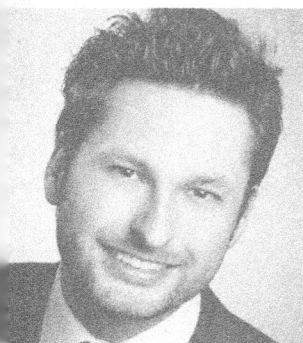
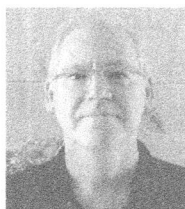
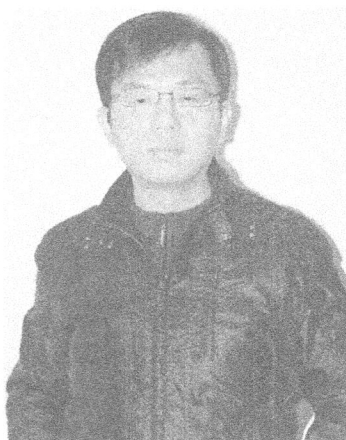

IntechOpen

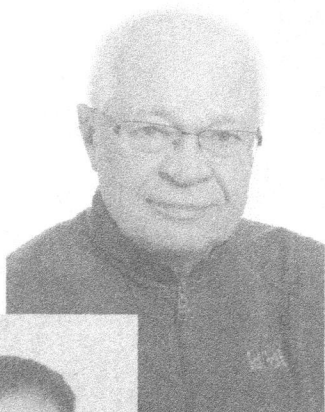
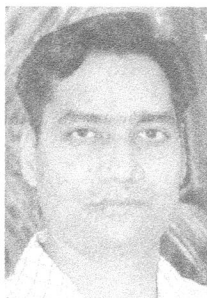
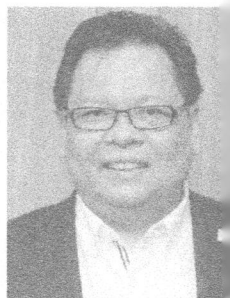
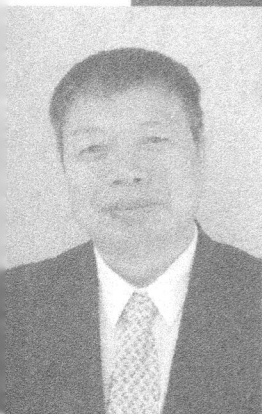
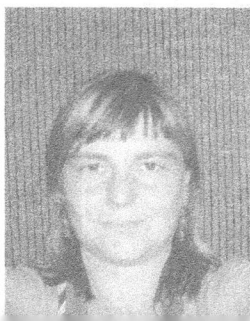
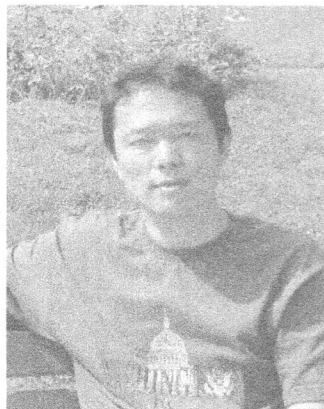

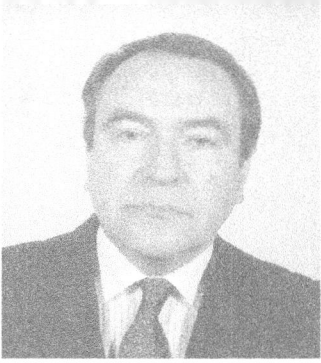

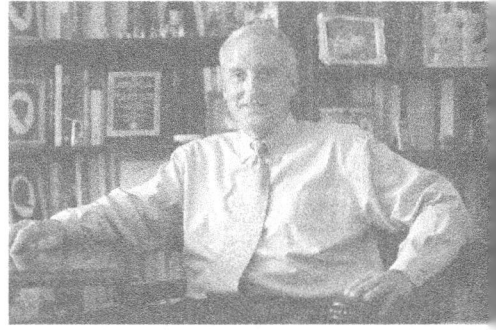

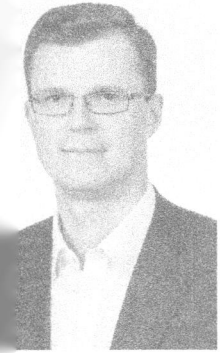

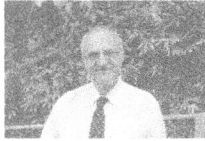

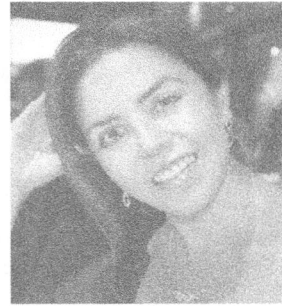

Supporting open minds since 2005

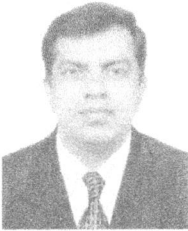

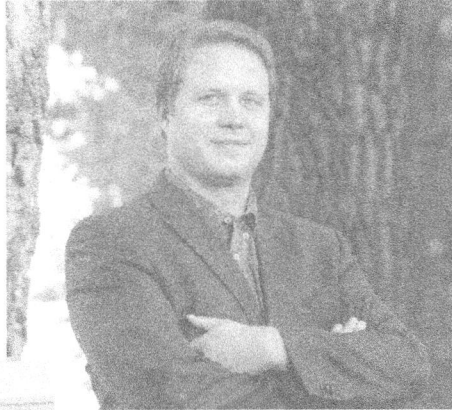

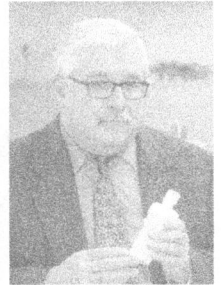

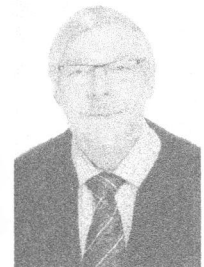

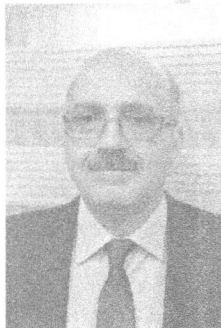

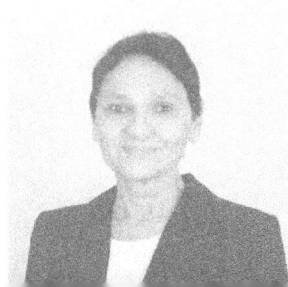

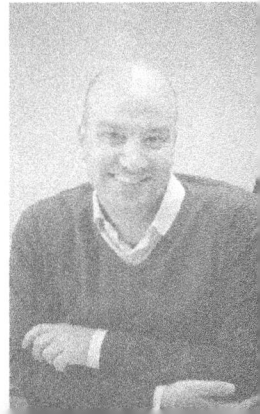

Prions – Some Physiological and Pathophysiological Aspects
http://dx.doi.org/10.5772/intechopen.74080
Edited by Ivo Nikolaev Sirakov

Contributors

Saima Zafar, Inga Zerr, Yannick Bailly, Audrey Ragagnin, Qili Wang, Aurélie Guillemain, Siaka Dole, Anne-Sophie Wilding, Valérie Demais, Cathy Royer, Anne-Marie Haeberlé, Nicolas Vitale, Stéphane Gasman, Nancy Grant, Keiji Uchiyama, Suehiro Sakaguchi, Ivo Nikolaev Sirakov

Notice

Statements and opinions expressed in the chapters are these of the individual contributors and not necessarily those of the editors or publisher. No responsibility is accepted for the accuracy of information contained in the published chapters. The publisher assumes no responsibility for any damage or injury to persons or property arising out of the use of any materials, instructions, methods or ideas contained in the book.

First published in London, United Kingdom, 2019 by IntechOpen
IntechOpen is the global imprint of INTECHOPEN LIMITED, registered in England and Wales, registration number: 11086078, The Shard, 25th floor, 32 London Bridge Street
London, SE19SG – United Kingdom
Printed in Croatia

British Library Cataloguing-in-Publication Data
A catalogue record for this book is available from the British Library

Additional hard copies can be obtained from orders@intechopen.com

Prions – Some Physiological and Pathophysiological Aspects
Edited by Ivo Nikolaev Sirakov
p. cm.
Print ISBN 978-1-78985-017-8
Online ISBN 978-1-78985-018-5

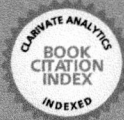

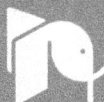

Meet the editor

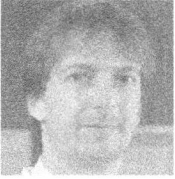

In 2005, Ivo Nikolaev Sirakov graduated in Veterinary Medicine in Sofia and in 2012, he received his PhD degree at the Bulgarian Food Safety Agency. He works as an assistant and Assistant Professor at the NRL "TSE" where he is responsible for diagnosis of TSEs by WB, IHC, and ELISA methods; sequencing of the sheep and goat prion protein gene; and a number of training programs that he has led in reference laboratories in the EU. He has participated as a government expert in discussions on TSE-related legislation in the EC. From 2013 to 2015, he was head of the NRL "Enzootic Bovine Leukosis" and a lecturer at the Medical University of Sofia. Since 2015, he works as an assistant and Head Assistant Professor at Department of "Medical Microbiology", MU -Sofia.

Contents

Chapter 1

Introductory Chapter: Prions

Ivo Nikolaev Sirakov

1. Introduction

The cellular prion protein (PrP^C) is expressed as a cell surface protein mainly in the central and peripheral nervous system, as well as in some cells and organs of the immune system (leukocytes and the spleen), the reproductive system (the testes and ovaries), and others, such as Peyer's patches in the intestinal tract, heart, lungs, and skeletal muscles, spreading to almost all parts of the body [1]. Prions were only relatively recently revealed to act as infectious agents although the diseases they cause have been known for a long time—initially attributed to toxic, genetic, and psychological factors and "unconventional viruses"—as our understanding of their mechanism evolved together with the methodological advancements.

The discovery that prions are infectious agents changed the concept of protein synthesis in modern biology and built a bridge between the genesis of infectious and genetic diseases.

The normal distribution of PrP^C in certain organs correlates with the pathogenesis route of some prion diseases, such as scrapie, Kuru, bovine spongiform encephalopathy (BSE), new variant Creutzfeldt-Jakob disease (vCJD), chronic wasting disease (CWD), and feline spongiform encephalopathy (FSE), probably acting as a "transformer and conductor" of the infectious isoform.

From a historical perspective, scrapie—as a disease of sheep—was a subject of discussion in the British parliament back in 1755; however, it was not until 1936 that Cullie and Chelle proved its contagious character by experimental infection [2]. Studies demonstrated genetic predisposition to development of the disease [3].

The disease bovine spongiform encephalopathy (BSE) was first identified and reproduced in 1986 in the United Kingdom [4]. It resulted from an incinerating technology introduced in the 1970s that worked at a lower disposal temperature and the supplementation of calf feed mixtures with meat-bone meal from scrapie sheep.

In Wisconsin, USA, in 1947, the disease transmissible mink encephalopathy (TME) was reported, arising from the use of sheep carcasses for food. Due to the cannibalism existing among minks and the passages through them, the etiological agent has undergone changes (e.g., it is nonpathogenic to mice) [2]. Another prion disease in animals is chronic wasting disease (CWD), which affects cervids including deer, elk, and moose. It was described by Williams and Young in 1980 [5], and no genetic determinant was detected for its development.

Feline spongiform encephalopathy (FSE) was first reported as a disease in members of family Felidae in a zoo in the UK [6] and in other carnivorous animals. Eventually, the infection was demonstrated to originate from BSE [7], the source of infection being contaminated food. BSE is also the etiological agent of diseases in Nyala, Kudu—exotic ungulate encephalopathy (EUE)—and Lemurs (NHP—BSE in nonhuman primates) [6, 8].

There is a direct relationship between the prion diseases in animals and humans due to the ability of BSE to jump the barrier between species (via contaminated food) and the emergence of a new variant of CJD in the UK in 1996 [9, 10] affecting mainly young people aged 27–35 years. The prions isolated from these patients are glycosylated at two sites (like BSE), and their gene encoding PrP has a characteristic homozygosity at codon 129 (methionine-methionine) [2].

Creutzfeldt–Jakob disease (CJD) was reported back in 1920 [11], and the elucidation of the etiology of Kuru (see below) prompted Gajdusek and coworkers to prove the infectious nature of this disease (CJD) by successfully transmitting it to chimpanzees and other species of monkeys. The disease may be manifested in several epidemic forms: iatrogenic CJD (iCJD) [12] resulting from surgical interventions (corneal grafting), use of contaminated electrodes in encephalography, sporadic CJD (sCJD) resulting from spontaneous mutations [11], and other TSE diseases associated with mutations in the coding gene, for example, familial or genetic f/gCJD [13], Gerstmann-Sträussler-Scheinker syndrome (GSS) [14], fatal familial insomnia (FFI) [15], sporadic fatal insomnia (sFI) [16], and variably protease-sensitive prionopathy (VPSPr) [17].

Kuru is an interesting form spread among the natives of the Fore linguistic group inhabiting the mountainous regions of Papua New Guinea. The disease was studied by Gajdusek and coworkers in the 1960s. Based on its similarity to scrapie and epidemiological, clinical, and pathohistological features [18], Gajdusek managed to reproduce the disease in chimpanzees [19]. The research proved that the disease is noncontagious but transmitted by a tribal funeral ritual in which the deceased one's relatives pay their respect by eating his/her undercooked brain [2].

In one way or another, all prion diseases in animals and humans are of social and economic importance. It is alarming that human activity—guided by economic, ritual, or other considerations—could trigger the evolution of a pathogen so that it progressively crosses the barrier between two species within just a few decades or turns into a strain characteristic of a specific species or ethnic group. This comes to demonstrate, in a negative perspective, how deep and strong an effect can unconscious human interference have on biological processes. The mechanisms underlying these processes, however, still remain largely unknown. That is why, to correctly unravel the pathogenic processes, it is also important to gain a deeper understanding of the normal role of the prion protein and the processes that accompany it. Hence, this book discusses the normal function of the prion protein (PrP^C) and its modulatory role in synaptic mechanisms. It describes the pathophysiological processes that accompany TSE, such as neurotoxicity, loss of anti-inflammatory protective function, and the mechanisms of neuronal death including prion-induced autophagy and apoptosis. In TSE, specifically there is accumulation of an isoform of the normal protein (PrP^{Sc}) in the cytoplasm of neurons. Thus, it is important to understand the mechanism underlying this process, which is also reviewed in this book. Another aspect outlined here is that some prion diseases show strain variations, which determine their development, demonstrating their key role in the development and progression of TSE.

Author details

Ivo Nikolaev Sirakov
Department of Medical Microbiology, Faculty of Medicine, Medical University of
Sofia, Sofia, Bulgaria

*Address all correspondence to: insirakov@gmail.com

IntechOpen

References

[1] Bendheim PE, Brown HR, Rudelli RD, Scala LJ, Goller NL, Wen GY, et al. Nearly ubiquitous tissue distribution of the scrapie agent precursor protein. Neurology. 1992;**42**:149

[2] Haralambiev H. Animal Viruses. A Short Virology Manual. Haskovo, Bulgaria: Pandora. 2002;**1**:141-151

[3] Hunter N, Cairns D, Foster J, Smith G, Goldman W, Donnelly K. Is scrapie a genetic disease? Evidence from scrapie free countries. Nature. 1997;**386**:137-137

[4] Wells GAH, Scott AC, Johnson CT, Gunning RF, Hancock RD, Jeffrey M, et al. A novel progressive spongiform encephalopathy in cattle. The Veterinary Record. 1987;**121**:419-420

[5] Williams ES, Young S. Chronic wasting disease of captive mule deer: A spongiform encephalopathy. Journal of Wildlife Diseases. 1980;**16**:89-98

[6] Kirkwood JK, Cunningham AA. Epidemiological observations on spongiform encephalopathies in captive wild animals in the British Isles. The Veterinary Record. 1994;**135**:296-303. DOI: 10.1136/vr.135.13.296

[7] Fraser H, Pearson GR, McConnell I, Bruce ME, Wyatt JM, Gruffydd-Jones TJ. Transmission of feline spongiform encephalopathy to mice. Veterinary Record. 1994;**134**(17):449

[8] Sigurdson CJ, Miller MW. Other animal prion diseases. British Medical Bulletin. 2003;**66**:199-212

[9] Will RG, Ironside JW, Zeidler M, Estibeiro K, Cousens SN, Smith PG, et al. A new variant of Creutzfeldt-Jakob disease in the UK. The Lancet. 1996;**347**(9006):921-925

[10] Bruce ME, Will RG, Ironside JW, McConnell I, Drummond D, Suttie A, et al. Transmissions to mice indicate that 'new variant' CJD is caused by the BSE agent. Nature. 1997;**389**(6650):498

[11] Creutzfeldt HG. U" ber eine eigenartige herdfo"rmige erkrankung des zentralnervensystems. Zeitschrift für die Gesamte Neurologie und Psychiatrie. 1920;**57**:1-19. DOI: 10.1007/BF02866081

[12] Duffy P, Wolf J, Collins G, DeVoe AG, Streeten B, Cowen D. Possible person-to-person transmission of Creutzfeldt-Jakob disease. The New England Journal of Medicine. 1974;**290**:692-693

[13] Kirschbaum WR. Zwei eigenartige erkrankung des zentralnervensystems nach Art der spatischen pseudosklerose (Jakob). Zeitschrift für die Gesamte Neurologie und Psychiatrie. 1924;**92**:175-220. DOI: 10.1007/BF02877841

[14] Adam JA, Crow TJ, Duchen LW, Scaravilli F, Spokes E. Familial cerebral amyloidosis and spongiform encephalopathy. Journal of Neurology, Neurosurgery & Psychiatry. 1982;**45**(1):37-45

[15] Lugaresi E, Medori R, Montagna P, Baruzzi A, Cortelli P, Lugaresi A, et al. Fatal familial insomnia and dysautonomia with selective degeneration of thalamic nuclei. The New England Journal of Medicine. 1986;**315**:997-1003. DOI: 10.1056/NEJM198610163151605

[16] Mastrianni JA, Nixon R, Layzer R, Telling GC, Han D, DeArmond SJ, et al. Prion protein conformation in a patient with sporadic fatal insomnia. The New England Journal of Medicine. 1999;**340**:1630-1638. DOI: 10.1056/NEJM199905273402104

[17] Gambetti P, Dong Z, Yuan J, Xiao X, Zheng M, Alshekhlee A, et al. A novel

human disease with abnormal prion protein sensitive to protease. Annals of Neurology. 2008;**63**:697-708. DOI: 10.1002/ana.21420

[18] Hadlow WJ. Scrapie and kuru. Lancet. 1959;**II**:289-290

[19] Gajdusek DC, Alpers M. Experimental transmission of a kuru-like syndrome to chimpanzees. Nature. 1966;**209**(5025):794

Chapter 2

Prion Proteins and Neuronal Death in the Cerebellum

Audrey Ragagnin, Qili Wang, Aurélie Guillemain, Siaka Dole,
Anne-Sophie Wilding, Valérie Demais, Cathy Royer,
Anne-Marie Haeberlé, Nicolas Vitale, Stéphane Gasman,
Nancy Grant and Yannick Bailly

Abstract

The cellular prion protein, a major player in the neuropathology of prion diseases, is believed to control both death and survival pathways in central neurons. However, the cellular and molecular mechanisms underlying these functions remain to be deciphered. This chapter presents cytopathological studies of the neurotoxic effects of infectious prions and cellular prion protein-deficiency on cerebellar neurons in wild-type and transgenic mice. The immunochemical and electron microscopy data collected in situ and ex vivo in cultured organotypic cerebellar slices indicate that an interplay between apoptotic and autophagic pathways is involved in neuronal death induced either by the infectious prions or by prion protein-deficiency.

Keywords: prion protein, Doppel, apoptosis, autophagy, cerebellum, mouse

1. Introduction

1.1 Prion diseases

Transmissible spongiform encephalopathies (TSEs) or "prion diseases" are fatal neurodegenerative disorders in humans (Creutzfeldt-Jakob disease (CJD), Gerstmann-Sträussler-Scheinker syndrome (GSS), variant CJD (vCJD), fatal familial insomnia (FFI) and kuru) and in animals (bovine spongiform encephalopathy (BSE), transmissible mink encephalopathy (TME), chronic wasting disease of cervids (CWD), camel prion disease (CPD), and scrapie of sheep and goats) [1–4]. Prevailing over a viral etiology, the conformational corruption of host-encoded cellular prion protein (PrP^c) by a pathogenic isoform (PrP^{TSE}) is now widely accepted as underlying prion transmission and pathogenesis in TSEs [5–7].

1.2 PrP^c functions

Prnp-knockout mice were generated in order to investigate the physiological functions of PrP^c. In either mixed C57BL/6 j x129/Sv(ev) (Zurich I, ZrchI, *Prnp*$^{ZH1/ZH1}$, [8]) or pure 129/Ola (Npu, Edinburgh, Edbg, [9]) or C57BL/6J (Zurich III, ZrchIII, *Prnp*$^{ZH3/ZH3}$, [10]) genetic backgrounds, the first *Prnp* null mouse strains produced were viable with no clear abnormality except for their resistance to prion infection [11] and absence of obvious neurodegeneration. Similar absence of neurodegeneration or histopathology resulted from depletion of neuronal PrP^c in adult conditional *Prnp*-knockout NFH-Cre/tg37 mice [12]. Thus, a physiological function of PrP^c that is essential for life seemed to be ruled out unless it is highly redundant or is compensated. Nevertheless, looking at different neuronal and other cell functions in PrP^c-ablated mice has revealed a number of differences that can be attributed to the physiological functions of PrP^c (see [13] for review).

PrP^c has been implicated in neurotransmission, olfaction, proliferation and differentiation of neural precursor cells, neuritic growth, neuronal homeostasis, cell signaling, cell adhesion, myelin maintenance, copper and zinc transport, as well as neuroprotection against toxic insults, such as oxidative stress and excitotoxicity (see [14, 15] for reviews). Increasing evidence links prion protein misfolding and accumulation to neurodegeneration in prion diseases. Accordingly, several nonexclusive mechanisms of prion-mediated neurotoxicity are currently under investigation (see [16] for review). PrP^c has been localized in three major sites: enriched in lipid rafts, anchored in the outer plasma membrane leaflet by its GPI tail [17], and intracellularly in the Golgi apparatus early and late endosomes [18, 19]. Since lipid rafts are pivotal microdomains for signal transduction, PrP^c is likely triggering intracellular signaling pathways [20, 21]. The first evidence that PrP^c might mediate extracellular signals was the caveolin-1-dependent coupling of PrP^c to the tyrosine-protein kinase Fyn [21]. From this pioneering work, accumulating data suggested that PrP^c functions as a "dynamic cell surface platform for the assembly of signaling molecules," partnering with other membrane proteins to transduce cellular signaling [22].

1.3 Synaptic PrP^c

Whereas, PrP^c is highly expressed in both neurons and glial cells of the CNS [19, 23, 24], it is preferentially localized in the pre- and postsynaptic terminals of neurons [19, 24, 25]. Immunocytochemical studies of primate and rodent brains [25, 26] including an EGFP-tagged PrP^c in transgenic mice, showed that PrP^c is enriched along axons and presynaptic terminals [27–29], and undergoes anterograde and retrograde transport [30, 31]. Such a synaptic targeting of PrP^c suggests that it could be involved in preserving synaptic structure and function. Indeed, synaptic dysfunction and loss are early prominent events in prion diseases [32, 33]. However, a functional role of PrP^c at synapses is not consistently supported by functional data and still remains contentious.

Insights into possible mechanisms by which PrP^c modulates synaptic mechanisms and neuronal excitability at a molecular level have been provided by the documented interactions of PrP^c with several ion channels including the voltage-gated calcium channels (VGCCs) [34], the N-methyl-D-aspartate glutamate receptors (NMDARs) [35] and the voltage-gated potassium channels Kv4.2 [36]. PrP^c has been shown to regulate NMDARs due to its affinity for copper that leads to inhibition of glutamate receptors and excitotoxicity [37, 38]. While interaction of PrP^c with these channels may account for some of its functions, a toxic response can also be activated when PrP^c misfolds. A structural change in cell surface PrP^c has been proposed to simultaneously disrupt NMDAR function and plasma membrane permeability, leading to dysregulation of ion homeostasis and neuronal death [39, 40]. PrP^c can also interact with kainate receptor subunits GluR6/7 [41], α-amino-3-hydroxy-5-methyl-4-isoxazolepropionic acid (AMPA) receptors subunits GluA1 and GluA2 [42, 43], and metabotropic glutamate receptors of group 1 mGluR1 and mGluR5 [44, 45]. PrP^c can interact with the β-amyloid peptide (Aβ) and the later [45, 46] is believed to underlie the Aβ oligomer-induced disruption of LTP in Alzheimer's disease [47]. Thus, PrP^c seems to behave as a cell surface receptor for synaptic oligomers of the Aβ peptide and, of other β-sheet-rich neurotoxic proteins [40].

1.4 PrP^{TSE}-related neurotoxicity in prion diseases

The histopathological signature of TSEs notably relies on the aggregation of PrP^{TSE}, vacuolation of the brain tissue, astrogliosis, and synaptic and neuronal loss. How neurons, the major targets of prions, die, remains a central question in prion diseases. The absence of neurodegenerative phenotypes after depletion of PrP^c suggests that neurotoxicity is not due to a loss of PrP^c function but rather results from a gain of toxicity upon its conversion to PrP^{TSE}, which then acts on the central nervous system (CNS) [48]. Although PrP^c is required for propagation of infectious prions and PrP^{TSE}-mediated toxicity [49], the mechanisms by which prions are lethal for neurons remain mostly unknown. Nevertheless, the endogenous PrP^c conversion has been shown to cause neuronal dysfunction and death, rather than PrP^{TSE} itself which does not seem to be directly neurotoxic. A precise understanding of the factors leading to neurotoxicity in prion infections is crucial to developing targeted therapies and investigating the role of PrP^c in neurons should provide insight.

The conformational conversion of PrP^c begins on the neuronal surface, where PrP^c interacts with exogenous PrP^{TSE}, and then proceeds within endogenous compartments suggesting that neurotoxicity may be triggered by PrP^c misfolding both at the cell surface and inside the cell. In both acquired and genetic prion diseases, intracellular PrP^c misfolding would ultimately alter synaptic proteostasis, either through an indirect unfolded protein response (UPR)-mediated mechanism [50], likely arising either from an impairment of the neuronal ubiquitin-proteasome system (UPS) [51], or a direct interference with secretory trafficking of PrP^c-interacting cargoes [52]. Common features associated with prion infections include Ca^{2+} dysregulation, release of reactive oxygen species, and induction of endoplasmic-reticulum (ER) stress, which has been recently suggested as an important player in pathogenesis [53]. Prion-infected mice show brisk activation of the UPR and specifically of the PERK pathway, resulting in eIF2α phosphorylation and suppression of translational initiation. PERK inhibition protects mice from prion neurotoxicity, confirming an important pathogenic role of ER stress [50]. Since UPR activation and/or increased eIF2α-P levels as well as UPS impairment are commonly seen in prion disorders and in Alzheimer's and Parkinson's diseases, translational control, and UPS stimulation strategies may offer a common therapeutic opportunity to prevent synaptic failure and neuronal loss in protein misfolding diseases [51, 54].

1.5 Loss of PrP^c anti-inflammatory protective function in prion disease

A protective role of PrP^c against a noxious insult mediated by the pro-inflammatory cytokine tumor necrosis factor-α (TNFα) has recently been demonstrated [55]. The α-secretase activity mediated by the TNFα-converting enzyme (TACE) was impaired at the surface of Fukuoka and 22L scrapie prion-infected neurons. Furthermore, the activity of 3-phosphoinositide-dependent kinase-1 (PDK1) which inactivates phosphorylation and caveolin-1-mediated internalization of TACE is increased in scrapie-infected neurons. PDK1 was shown to be controlled by RhoA-associated coiled-coil containing kinases (ROCK) which favored the PrP^{TSE} production. In these neurons, exacerbated ROCK activity overstimulated PDK1 activity which canceled the neuroprotective α-cleavage of PrP^c by TACE α-secretase, physiologically precluding PrP^{TSE} production. Inhibition of ROCK lowered PrP^{TSE} in prion-infected cells as well as in the brain of prion-diseased mice which had extended lifespans [56]. Indeed, the dysregulation of TACE resulted in PrP[TSE] accumulation and reduced the shedding of TNFα receptor type 1 (TNFR1) from the neuronal plasma membrane. Inversely, inhibition of PDK1 *in vitro* promoted TACE localization at the plasma membrane, restoring TACE-dependent α-secretase activity and shedding of PrP[c] and TNFR1, thereby attenuating PrP[TSE]-induced neurotoxicity. Similarly, inhibition or siRNA-mediated silencing of PDK1 extended survival and reduced motor impairment of scrapie-diseased mice [55]. Mechanistically, PrP[c] coupling to the NADPH oxidase-TACE α-secretase signaling pathway limits the sensitivity of recipient cells to TNFα by promoting TACE-mediated cleavage of TNFα receptors (TNFRs) and the release of soluble TNFRs. PrP[c] expression was further shown to be necessary for maintaining TACE α-secretase at the plasma membrane and its TNFR shedding activity. The loss of PrP[c] provoked TACE internalization, canceling TACE-mediated cleavage of TNFR. This rendered PrP[c]-depleted cells and *Prnp*-knockout mice highly vulnerable to pro-inflammatory TNFα insult. Thus, abnormal trafficking and activity of TACE in prion diseases likely originates from a loss of PrP[c] cytoprotective function [57].

Synaptolysis is believed to initiate the neurodegeneration arising after a decrease in depolarization-induced calcium transients that progressively impairs glutamate release [34]. However, although cytoskeletal disruption in dendritic spines plays a major role in neuronal dysfunction, neither changes in postsynaptic densities and presynaptic compartment nor disruption of afferent innervation have been systematically observed, suggesting that even at terminal stages of the disease neuronal loss may not result from deafferentation as previously proposed in the hippocampus and cerebellum of scrapie-infected mice [33, 58, 59]. Thus, neuronal vulnerability to pathological protein misfolding appears to be more strongly dependent than previously thought, on the structure and function of target neurons.

Recent investigations of scrapie pathogenesis in the mouse cerebellum revealed an early upregulation of tumor necrosis factor-α receptor type 1 (TNFR1), a key mediator of neuroinflammation at the membrane of astrocytes enveloping Purkinje cell (PC) excitatory synapses already at the preclinical stage of the disease before PrP[22L] precipitation, GFAP astrogliosis, and PC death [59]. The contribution of perisynaptic astrocytes to prion pathogenesis through TNFR1 upregulation remains to be clarified and, although the cell types responsible for PrP[22L] production in the cerebellum are still uncertain, these data suggest a critical role for astrocytes in prion pathogenesis.

2. Mechanisms of neuronal death in prion diseases

Despite the overall advances made in this field during the last decades, the sequence of cellular and molecular events leading to neuronal cell demise in TSEs remains obscure. At present, neuronal cell death can be envisioned as resulting from several parallel, interacting, or sequential pathways involving protein processing and proteasome dysfunction [60], oxidative stress [61], inflammation [55] apoptosis, and autophagy [62]. The repertoire of pathways that lead to neuronal death is however limited [63]. In TSEs, apoptosis is the most popular theory of cell death but is not convincingly documented. In all cases, the probable disruption of both neuronal metabolism and circuits generates a pro-apoptotic signal for neurons. In addition to disruption of cellular proteostasis, UPS dysfunction may lead to neurotoxicity by activating pro-apoptotic pathways. PrP[TSE] aggresomes can associate with pro-apoptotic factors such as vimentin and caspases [60]. On the other hand, autophagy has been reported in TSEs, but its role in prion disease pathology is not well established [64]. However, the extensive synaptic autophagy observed

in prion diseases [65] has been proposed to contribute to overall synaptic degeneration, a major precocious pathological feature leading to neuronal death in TSEs.
This chapter reports recent biochemical and cytopathological studies investigating
the involvement of apoptosis and autophagy in neuronal loss induced by infectious
prions as well as by PrP^c-deficiency in the mouse cerebellum.

Among TSEs, scrapie is a natural ovine prion disease widely studied in mouse
models using murine-adapted prion strains (22L, ME7) that, akin to natural prion
strains, differ in their rate of disease progression (i.e., duration of the incubation
period), as well as the extent and regional pattern of brain histopathology [66, 67].
For example, the characteristic of a prion strain mostly relies on specific biochemical
properties related to PrP^{TSE} misfolding. The variable susceptibility of neuronal types to
prion infection also emerges as another critical parameter that underlies the complex
mechanisms of prion pathogenesis [54, 68, 69] and affects PrP^{TSE} progression along
defined anatomical routes [70]. The cellular and molecular mechanisms involved in
targeting PrP^{TSE} to specific neuronal populations [33, 71, 72] and neuron-to-neuron
spreading of prions in the CNS remain elusive [73].

In several prion diseases, the cerebellum is a preferential prion target for scrapie
[74–78], also observed in Creutzfeldt-Jakob disease (CJD) cases [79–87]. Cerebellar
circuits are exquisitely patterned and the expression patterns of zebrins in PCs define
a topographical map of genetically determined zones controlling sensory-motor
behavior [88, 89]. Subsets of PCs expressing zebrins alternate with subsets of zebrin-
free PCs, thus forming complementary stripes of biochemically distinct PCs [88]. The
most comprehensively studied zonal marker is zebrin II/aldolase C (ZII/AldC) [90].
The expression of ZII/AldC by itself, however, is not sufficient to recapitulate the full
complexity of the cerebellar cortex because of the many other PC subtypes [91, 92].

In a recent study [59], the parasagittal compartmentation of the cerebellar
cortex restricted 22L scrapie pathogenesis, including PrP^{22L} accumulation, PC
neurodegeneration, and gliosis. Indeed, PCs displayed a differential, subtype-
specific vulnerability to 22L prions with zebrin-expressing PCs being more resistant
to prion toxicity, whereas in stripes where PrP^{22L} accumulated most zebrin-deficient
PCs were lost and spongiosis was accentuated (**Figure 1**). Although this banding
pattern of PrP^{22L} accumulation is most likely delineated by structural constraints
of compartmentation, different biochemical properties of PC subpopulations may
well determine their differential resistance to scrapie prions.

2.1 Prion-induced apoptosis

2.1.1 Apoptotic pathways in prion-infected neurons

The mechanism of prion neurotoxicity requires neuronal expression of PrP^c
and is based on the subversion of its normal function triggered by an interaction
with PrP^{TSE} at the cell surface, thereby transducing a toxic signal into the cell.
Nevertheless, this has been challenged by the discovery of a monomeric, highly
α-helical form of PrP^c with strong *in vitro* and *in vivo* neurotoxicity that elicits
autophagy and apoptosis with a molecular signature similar to that observed in
prion-infected animal brains [93]. This toxic PrP (TPrP) killed PrP-deficient
neurons *in vitro* suggesting that a PrP-derived toxic signal can be generated within
neurons independently of endogenous membrane-bound PrP^c. Indeed, postnatal
ablation of PrP^c expression in neurons reversed neurodegeneration and affected
disease progression in mice even though glial replication was maintained and PrP^{TSE}
accumulated [94]. Thus, prion pathogenesis is governed by both cell-autonomous
mechanisms responsible for cellular dysfunction and neurodegeneration and
noncellular-autonomous mechanisms propagating prion spread [95].

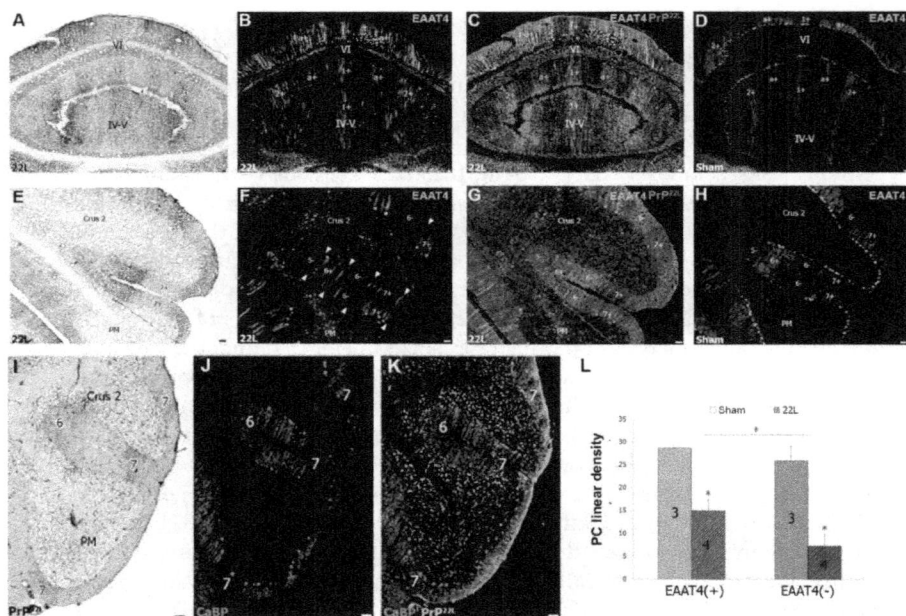

Figure 1.
*Banding pattern of PrP^{22L}, EAAT4 zebrin and PC loss in the EAAT4-eGFP mouse cerebellum **A–H**. The pattern of PrP^{22L} deposits (immunoperoxidase (immunoHRP) in A and E is artificially visualized in red in C and G) correlated with the banding pattern of the zebrin excitatory amino acid transporter 4 (EAAT4-eGFP, green in B, F) in merged PrP^{22L}-EAAT4 images C and G in the cerebellar vermis (A–C) and hemispheres (E–G) infected with 22L ic. (clinical stage 145 dpi). D, H. EAAT4-eGFP PCs in the same regions of the vermis (D) and hemisphere (H) of a noninfected EAAT4-eGFP mouse as shown in the cerebellum of the 22L-infected EAAT4-eGFP mouse (A–G). The zebrin bands are numbered according to the current nomenclature in A–K and indicated by arrowheads in F. **I–K**. In the cerebellum infected icb. (preclinical stage), two bands of PrP^{22L} deposits (6 and 7) are visualized by immunoHRP in I and artificially visualized in green in K. These cross crus2 and paramedian lobule (PM) and display a marked loss of CaBP-immunofluorescent PCs (red). Scale bars = 50 μm. **L**. Quantitative analysis of EAAT4-expressing and -nonexpressing PCs in the cerebellum of EAAT4-eGFP mice infected i.c. (clinical stage). The EAAT4-nonexpressing PCs are more sensitive to 22L toxicity. *$p < 0.05$. The number of mice analyzed is indicated on the bars in the graph.*

Endoplasmic-reticulum stress has recently been implicated in an apoptotic regulatory pathway activated by changes in Ca^{2+} homeostasis or accumulation of aggregated proteins. In both these situations, Ca^{2+} is released and caspase-12 is activated [96]. ER stress and caspase-12 activation have been identified in prion-infected N2a cells as well as in the brains of prion-diseased mice and CJD patients [97]. The synaptic dysfunction and neuronal death caused by PrP^{TSE} accumulation via dysregulation of the Ca^{2+}-sensitive phosphatase calcineurin (CaN) provides further evidence of the role of ER stress and Ca^{2+} homeostasis in prion-induced neurodegeneration [98]. The increase in Ca^{2+} cytosolic levels following hyperactivation of CaN dysregulates the pro-apoptotic Bcl-2-associated death promoter (Bad), and the transcription factor cAMP response element-binding (CREB). Dephosphorylated Bad interacts with Bax causing mitochondrial stress and apoptosis while dephosphorylated CREB cannot translocate into the nucleus to regulate the transcription of synaptic proteins, resulting in synaptic loss [99].

2.1.2 Mitochondrial apoptosis in prion-infected cerebellar neurons

PrP^c has recently been suggested to participate in anti-apoptotic and anti-oxidative processes by interacting with the stress inducible protein 1 (STI-1) to regulate superoxide dismutase (SOD) activation [100]. The PrP^c octapeptide repeat region contains a B-cell-lymphoma 2 (Bcl-2) homology domain 2 (BH2) of the family of apoptosis regulating Bcl-2 proteins involved in the anti-apoptotic function of Bcl-2. A direct interaction between PrPc and the C-terminus of anti-apoptotic Bcl-2 has also been found [101, 102]. In addition, the third helix of PrP^c impaired the BAX conformation changes required for apoptosis activation suggesting that PrP^c may assure the neuroprotective function of Bcl-2 [103]. Along this line, $Prnp^{0/0}$ neurons were more susceptible to apoptotic stimuli such as serum deprivation than their wild-type counterparts, whereas they were rescued by PrP^c or Bcl-2 expression [104, 105]. PrP^c also protected primary neurons against BAX-dependent apoptosis. Furthermore, transgenic expression of *Bax* or *Bax* and *Prnp* indicated that *Prnp* impairs *Bax*-dependent neuronal death [106].

Activation of the mitochondrial apoptotic pathway was observed when primary neurons were exposed to aggregated neurotoxic peptides like PrP106-126 or recombinant mutant PrP [107–109]. Apoptotic neuronal death demonstrated by activation of several caspases and DNA fragmentation is evident in natural prion diseases as well as in experimental models of TSEs [76, 110, 111]. In the cerebellum, apoptotic features have been observed in granule cells in CJD patients [112, 113] as well as in mice experimentally infected with CJD [111] and scrapie strains 301V, 87V, 22A [76], 79A [110], M1000/Fukuoka-1 [114], 127S [115], 22L, 139A, and RML [116, 117]. More recently, activation of caspase-3 was found in PCs of 22L-infected mice [59]. However, cerebral upregulation of the pro-apoptotic factor BAX has been reported in some cases of scrapie-infected rodents [116, 118], whereas no changes in clinical illness and neuropathology could be detected in the brain of Bax-deficient mice infected with 6PB1 mouse-adapted BSE prions [119]. This suggested that BAX-mediated cell death is not involved in the pathological mechanism induced by BSE. Nevertheless, BAX is known to be involved in neuronal death in Tg(PG14) [120] and Ngsk $PrnP^{0/0}$ [121] murine models of PrP-deficiency-linked diseases. In these cases, neuronal death is restricted to cerebellar neurons that are known to undergo BAX and BCL2-dependent apoptosis in other abnormal conditions [122, 123]. This led us to further investigate the involvement of intrinsic mitochondrial apoptotic pathways in a cerebellotropic prion disease such as the 22L scrapie. For this purpose, the pathogenesis of 22L scrapie in the brain of *Bax*-KO ($Bax^{-/-}$) mice [124] and in mice expressing a human Bcl-2 transgene [125] was analyzed. Clinical signs of 22L scrapie (mainly ataxia) were similar to those previously described for C57Bl/6 mice [126]. $Bax^{-/-}$ and HuBcl-2 mice infected by either intraperitoneal (ip.) or intracerebellar (icb.) route displayed ataxia 10–15 days sooner than wild-type mice. Survival times however, were similar in all genotypes (i.e., 223 dpi ip. and 129 dpi icb.). whereas 22L induced more severe cerebellar spongiosis via the icb. route than the ip. route, similar lesion profiles [71] were induced by 22L ip. in the brain of $Bax^{-/-}$ and wild-type mice and lesion profiles were not different in the brain of $Bax^{-/-}$, HuBcl-2 and wild-type mice infected with 22L icb. (**Figure 2**). Anatomopathological analysis of the cerebral and cerebellar cortices of the 22L-diseased $Bax^{-/-}$ and HuBcl-2 mice did not reveal any modified patterns of vacuolation, astrogliosis, and PrP^{22L} deposits irrespective of the inoculation route. Synaptophysin and calcium-binding protein (CaBP) immunohistochemistry also revealed severe synapse and PC loss in all cases (**Figure 3**). Finally, quantitative analysis of the cerebellar granule cells immunolabeled for the nuclear marker NeuN revealed a significant loss of neurons in all genotypes infected by the icb. route (**Figure 4**). Surprisingly, no significant difference could be detected between $Bax^{-/-}$ and wild-type mice infected by the icb. route, whereas HuBcl-2 mice whose granule cells are rescued from developmental cell death [127] lost more granule cells than wild-type and $Bax^{-/-}$ mice (**Figure 4**). These data indicate that neither suppression of *Bax* nor overexpression of Bcl-2 protected cerebellar neurons from 22L scrapie-induced neurotoxicity. Thus, the granule cell

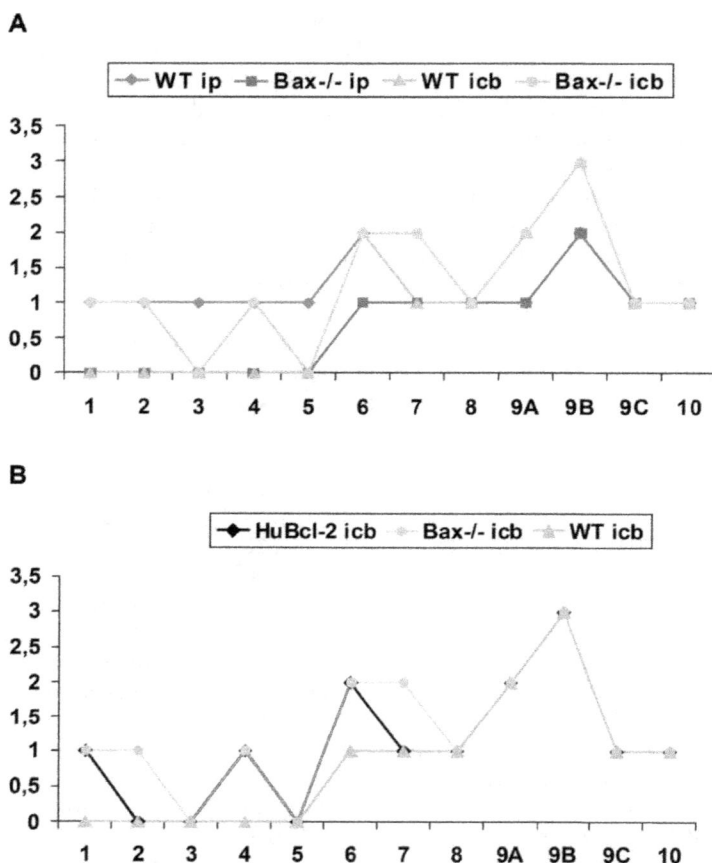

A

B

Figure 2.
*Spongiosis lesion profiles in the brain of wild-type (WT), Bax$^{-/-}$ and HuBcl-2 mice infected ip. and icb. with the 22L scrapie prion strain. **A**. Very similar lesion profiles were induced by 22L scrapie ip. in Bax$^{-/-}$ and WT mice. 22L induced more severe cerebellar spongiosis via the icb. route than via the ip. route. 1: cingulate and 2nd motor cortices, 2: lateral and medial septum, 3: caudate putamen, 4: retrosplenial cortex, 5: hippocampus, 6: thalamus, 7: hypothalamus, 8: superior colliculus, 9A: cerebellar molecular layer, 9B: cerebellar granular layer, 9C: cerebellar white matter, 10: medulla. **B**. Very similar lesion profiles were induced by 22L scrapie icb. in Bax$^{-/-}$, HuBcl-2 and WT mice.*

and PC death induced by 22L scrapie does not seem to involve BAX and cannot be counteracted by overexpression of the anti-apoptotic factor BCL-2. However, cleaved caspase-3 and -9 were observed in the brains of Bax$^{-/-}$ mice, suggesting that apoptosis may occur through (an) alternative mechanism(s) in TSEs of infectious origin. Indeed, apoptotic features have been reported in the brain of wild-type mice infected with RML, in the absence of Bax upregulation [116], while other proteins involved in cell death including those associated with the mitochondrial inner membrane, the UPS and the endoplasmic-reticulum-associated protein degradation (ERAD) pathway [128] were upregulated.

2.1.3 Prion-induced neuronal death in cerebellar organotypic slice cultures (COCS)

In the recently developed prion cerebellar organotypic slice culture (COCS) assay, progressive spongiform neurodegeneration that closely reproduce features of prion disease can be induced *ex vivo* [117, 129]. Infecting COCS with three different scrapie strains (RML, 22L, 139A) produced three distinct patterns of prion protein

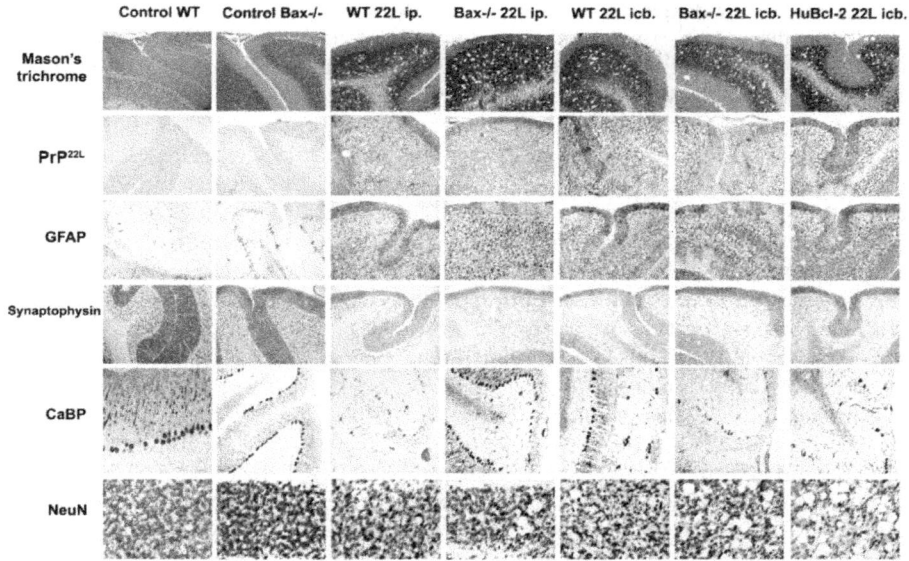

Figure 3.
Anatomopathology of 22L scrapie ip. and icb. in the cerebellum of WT, Bax⁻/⁻ and HuBcl-2 mice. Neither Bax knockout nor HuBcl-2 overexpression modified vacuolation (Mason's trichrome), astrogliosis (GFAP immunoHRP) and PrP²²ᴸ accumulation (PrP immunoHRP) patterns in the cerebellar cortex of the 22L ip. and icb. infected Bax⁻/⁻ and HuBcl-2 mice compared to the WT mice. Synaptophysin and CaBP reveal respectively synapse and PC loss in the cerebellum of all mice. Loss of Neun-immunostained GCs is also prominent in the cerebellum of the WT, Bax⁻/⁻ and HuBcl-2 infected icb., yet seemed less pronounced in the mice infected ip.

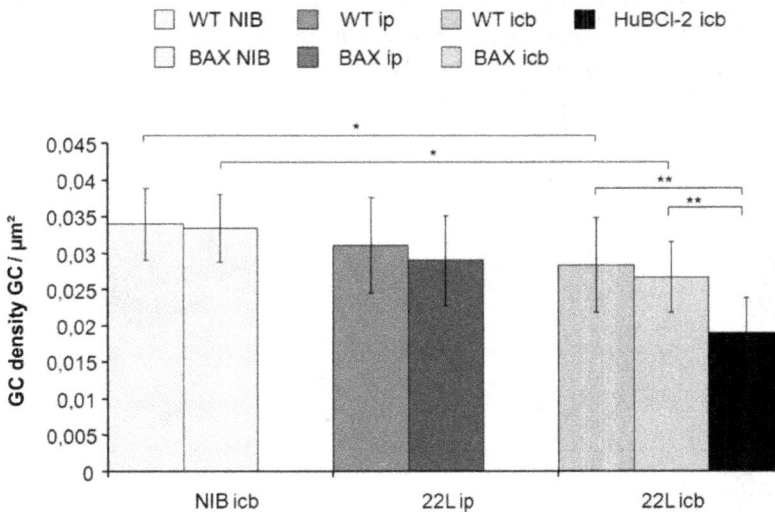

Figure 4.
Quantitative analysis of cerebellar GCs immunostained for the nuclear marker NeuN revealed a significant loss of neurons in all genotypes infected icb., but not ip. $^*p < 0.05$; $^{**}p < 0.01$. Whereas Bax⁻/⁻ and WT mice lost a similar amount of GCs, the HuBcl-2 mice lost more GCs than the WT and Bax⁻/⁻ mice. NIB, noninfected brain homogenate.

deposition accompanied by salient features of prion disease pathogenesis such as severe neuronal loss, a pro-inflammatory response, and typical neuropathological changes (spongiform vacuolation, tubulovesicular structures, neuronal dystrophy, and gliosis). Neurodegeneration did not occur when PrP was genetically removed from neurons and was abrogated by compounds known to antagonize prion replication. Also, calpain inhibitors, but not caspase inhibitors, prevented neurotoxicity and fodrin cleavage; whereas, prion replication was unimpeded indicating that inhibiting calpain uncouples prion replication and neurotoxicity. These data validate the COCS as a powerful model system that faithfully reproduces many morphological hallmarks of prion infections and shows that prion neurotoxicity in cerebellar granule cells is calpain-dependent but caspase-independent.

Furthermore, significant spine loss and altered dendritic morphology, analogous to that seen *in vivo* were induced by RML scrapie in COCS [130], while the deposition pattern and subcellular distribution of PrP^{22L} (i.e., granular deposits associated with neurons, astrocytes, and microglia but not PCs in the neuropil of the PC and molecular layers [131]), closely resembled that observed *in vivo* [59].

Following infection of COCS from C57Bl6/J, ZH-I Prnp$^{0/0}$, and Tga20 PrP-over-expressing mice with brain homogenate from C57Bl6/J infected intracerebrally (ic.) with either 22L or 139A scrapie prions, PrP^{22L} and PrP^{139A} accumulation could be detected on histoblots from wild-type and Tga20 COCS, respectively, 30 and 20 days post infection (dpi), but not on histoblots from ZH-I mice (**Figure 5**). Furthermore, quantitative analysis of PCs in these COCs indicated that a severe loss of neurons was induced by 22L prions in wild-type slices at 30 dpi (22 ± 2 surviving PCs/slice) and in Tga20 slices at 20 dpi (293 ± 68 surviving PCs) as well as by 139A prions in wild-type slices at 30 dpi (145 ± 63 surviving PCs/slice) and in Tga20 slices at 20 dpi (191 ± 31 surviving PCs/slice) compared to noninfected control COCS (220 ± 27 surviving PCs/slice in wild-type slices and 357 ± 71 surviving PCs/slice in Tga20 slices) (**Figure 6**). At 30 dpi, the trilaminar organization of the cerebellar cortex was evident in noninfected COCs, which did not exhibit any clear ultrastructural modifications (**Figure 7**). Nevertheless, numerous vacuoles, autophagosomes, and lysosomes had formed in granule cells infected by 22L and 139A (**Figure 8**). In diseased PCs, autophagosomes with double membranes and rough endoplasmic reticulum (Nissl bodies) formed compartmented organelles of various sizes (1–10 compartments) resembling different stages leading to multivesicular vacuoles (**Figure 9**). Although further investigations are necessary, these ultrastructural

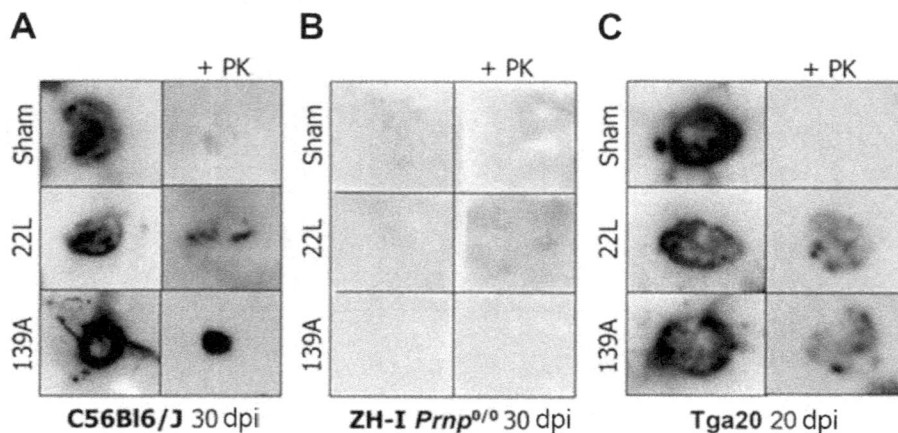

Figure 5.
Histoblots of cultured organotypic cerebellar slices (COCS) infected with the 22L and 139A scrapie strains. PrP^Sc was detected in histoblots of noninfected (sham) COCS from WT C57Bl6/J (A) and Tga20 PrP-overexpressing (C), but not PrP-deficient ZH-I PrnP^{0/0} (B) mice. PrP^Sc was completely digested by proteinase K (PK) in these COCS. After 30 and 20 days postinfection (dpi), PK revealed undigested PrP^{22L} and PrP^{139A} respectively in the WT and Tga20, but not ZH-I Prnp^{0/0} infected COCS.

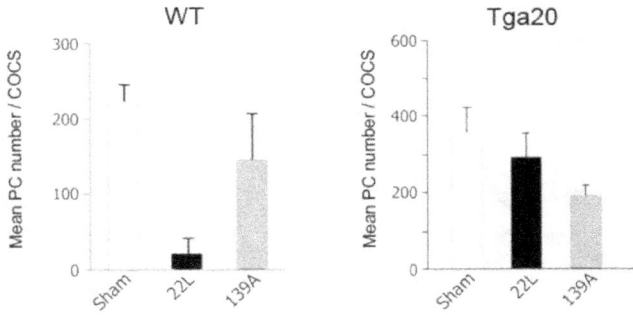

Figure 6.
Mean numbers of CaBP-immunofluorescent PCs in WT and Tga20 COCS noninfected (sham) and infected with 22L and 139A scrapie prions at 30 dpi.

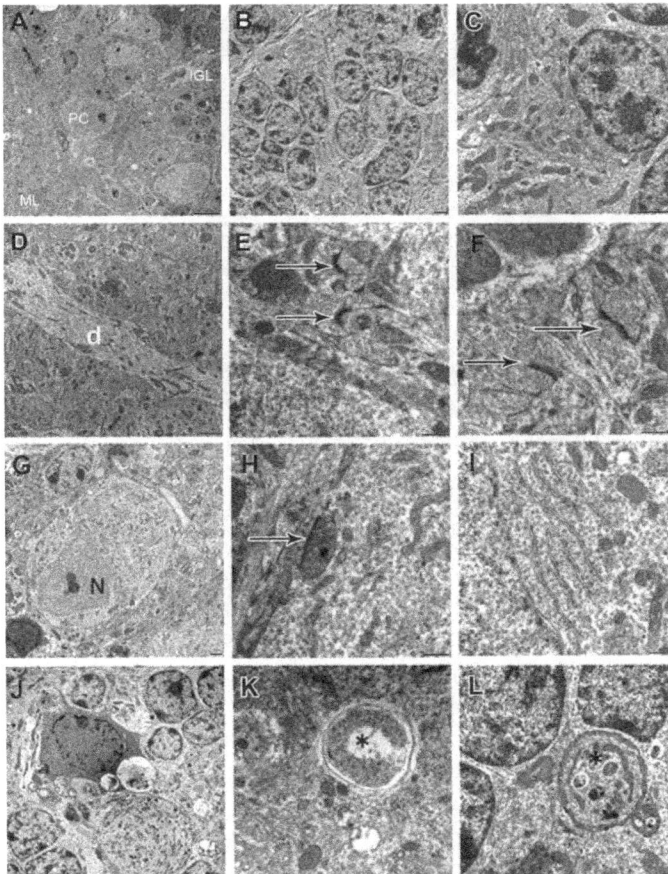

Figure 7.
Ultrastructural features of the C57Bl6/J mouse cerebellar cortex in noninfected COCS after 30 DIV. A. Laminar organization of the cerebellar cortex with PC at the interface between internal granular layer (IGL) and molecular layer (ML). B. Granule cells in the IGL. C. IGL neuropil. D. PC dendrite (d) in the ML neuropil. E, F. Asymmetrical synapses (arrows) on interneurons dendrites (E) and PC spines (F). G. PC. N, PC nucleus. H. A smooth saccule (arrow) typically separates a mitochondrion from the plasma membrane in the PC neuroplasm. I. Nissl body in the PC neuroplasm. J. Degenerated cell with electron-dense vacuolated cytoplasm. K. Autophagic digestion of a mitochondrion (*). L. Autophagic profiles in a PC axon (*). Scale bars = 10 μm in A, 2 μm in B–D, G, J, 500 nm in E, F, H, I, K, L.

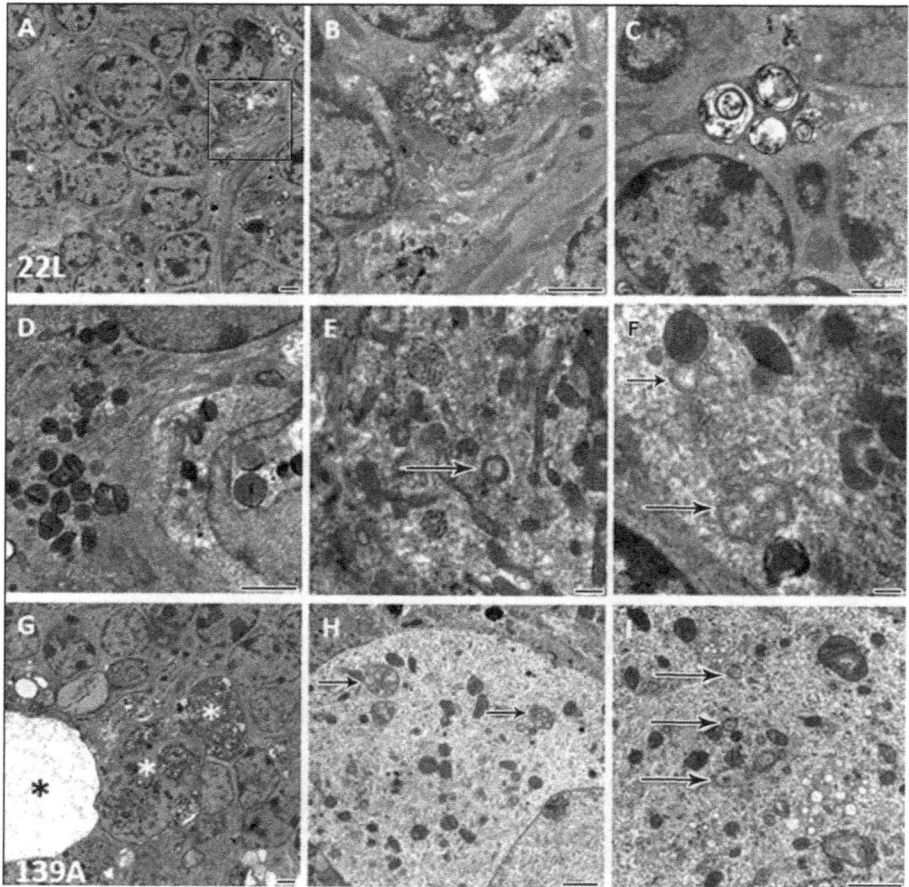

Figure 8.
*Cytopathology of the C57Bl6/J mouse cerebellar cortex in COCS infected with 22L (A–F) and 139A (G–L) scrapie prions at 30 dpi. **A**. IGL. **B–D**. Autophagic profiles in the IGL neuropil. **B**. Magnification of the inset in A. **D**. Electron-dense lysosomes. **E, F**. Various stages of ER-derived reticulated organelles (arrows) in the neuroplasm of a PC. **G**. Neurodegenerating profiles (*) in the IGL neuropil. **H, I.** PC neuroplasm containing different stages of ER-derived reticulated organelles (arrows) and vacuoles. Scale bars = 2 μm in A–D, G–I, 500 nm in E, F.*

alterations were not observed in noninfected slices suggesting that a specific effect of prions links prion-induced ER stress to this morphological ER modification.

2.2 Prion-induced autophagy

Autophagy and apoptosis are activated in many neurodegenerative diseases featured by ubiquitinated misfolded proteins. In neurons, the degradation of abnormal proteins such as α-synuclein in Parkinson's disease, β-amyloid peptide in Alzheimer's disease (AD), or PrP in TSEs occurs by autophagy [14, 132–135]. These cardinal proteins contribute to synaptic dysregulation and altered organelles leading to apoptosis. The neurodegenerating neurons exhibit robust accumulation of cytosolic autophagosomes (see [14] for review, **Figure 10**) suggesting a dysregulation of the autophagic flux resulting from autophagic stress, due to an imbalance between protein synthesis and degradation [136]. Autophagy reduces intraneuronal aggregates and slows down the progression of clinical disease in experimental models of AD [137–139] and prion diseases [140, 141]. Thus, dysregulation of the autophagic

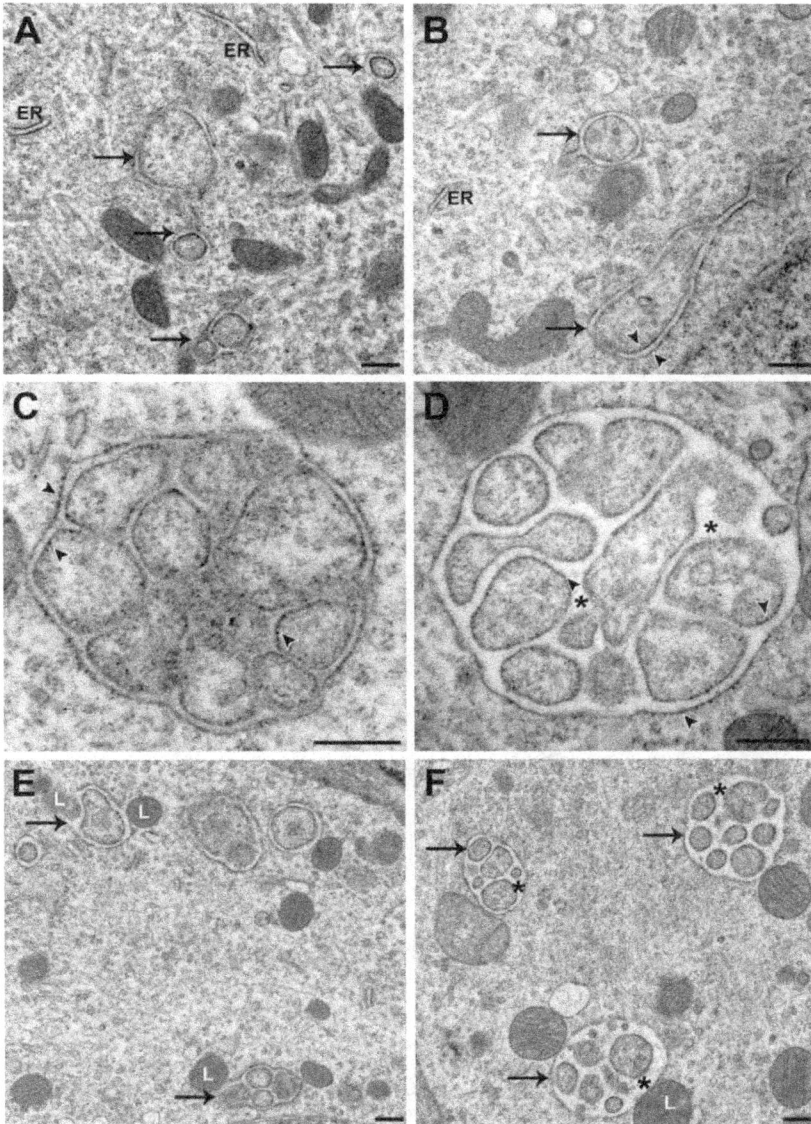

Figure 9.
*Cytopathological formation and evolution of ER-derived profiles in PCs of COCS infected with 139A scrapie prions at 30 dpi. **A, B**. Reticulation and sequestration of neuroplasm by ER saccules forming small double-membrane vesicles (arrows) containing ribosome-like particles (arrowheads in B) on both external and internal faces. ER, endoplasmic reticulum. **C, D**. Large compartmented ER-derived organelles which still display membrane-bound ribosomes (arrowheads). **C**. High magnification of **Figure 8H**. **D**. See the enlargement between membranes (*). **E**. Fusion (arrows) of small ER-derived double-membraned vacuoles with lysosomes (L). **F**. Large ER-derived double-membraned vacuoles with enlarged intermembrane space (*) transforming into multivesicular vacuoles (arrows). Scale bars = 500 nm.*

flux impairs the elimination of misfolded proteins and damaged organelles which then accumulate in the cytoplasm and contribute to cell dysfunction and death [142].

Together, spongiform vacuolation of the neuropil, synaptolysis, accompanied by neuronal cell loss and gliosis constitute the classical neuropathological quartet of TSEs. The typical "spongiform vacuoles" are believed to result from autophagy and develop within neuronal elements, myelinated axons, and myelin sheaths

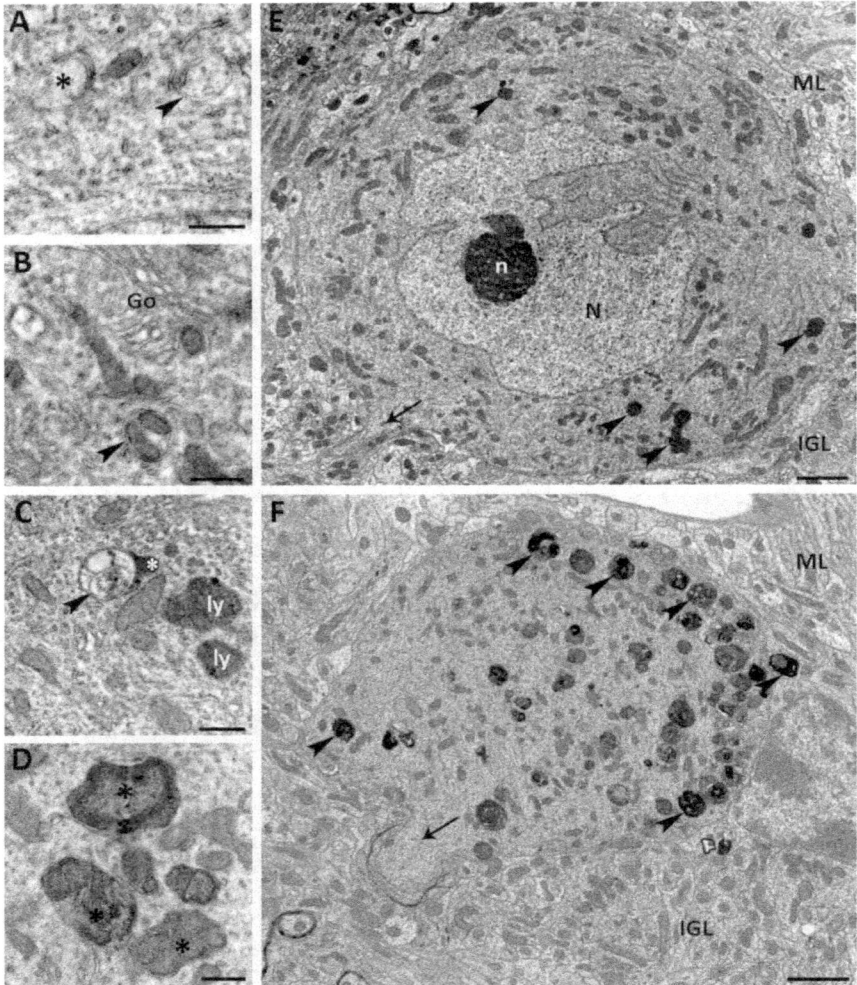

Figure 10.
*Autophagy in PCs of 4.5 (A–E) and 12 (F) month-old control Bax$^{+/+}$; Prnp$^{+/+}$ (E) and Bax$^{-/-}$;Ngsk Prnp$^{o/o}$ (A–D, F) mice. Ultrastructural autophagic stages from phagophores to autolysosomes. **A.** Phagophore (*) and double-membraned autophagosome (arrowhead). **B.** Sequestration of two mitochondria in an autophagosome (arrowhead). **Go**, Golgi dichtyosome. **C.** Fusion of an autophagosome (arrowhead) with a lysosome (*). Ly, lysosomes. **D.** Autolysosomes (*). A–D. Scale bars = 500 nm. **E.** The somato-dendritic cytoplasm of this control Bax$^{+/+}$; Prnp$^{+/+}$ PC contains a few lysosomes and lipofuchsin bodies (arrowheads). N, nucleus; n, nucleolus. **F.** Autophagic PC with numerous autophagic organelles (arrowheads) accumulating in the neuroplasm. ML, molecular layer. IGL, internal granular layer. E, F. Arrows show PC axon. Scale bars = 2 μm.*

[143, 144]. Autophagic vacuoles are increased in prion-diseased neurons [64, 65, 145], and the scrapie responsive gene 1 (SRG1) protein is overexpressed and bound to neuronal autophagosomes in the brain of scrapie- and BSE-infected animals and CJD-diseased humans [146, 147]. In addition, LC3-II, a marker of autophagosomes is increased in the cytosol of neurons in scrapie-infected hamsters and CJD- and FFI-diseased patients.

Recent evidence indicated that PrP^c, but not truncated PrP devoid of the N-terminal octapeptide repeat region, exerts a negative control on the induction of autophagy [148]. Thus, the loss or subversion of PrP^c function resulting from prion infection may upregulate autophagy in diseased neurons [16]. While autophagy-inducing agents increased cellular clearance of PrP^{TSE} [149–151], blocking the fusion of autophagosomes with lysosomes allowed visualization of PrP^{TSE} in the autophagosomes suggesting that degradation of endosomal PrP^{TSE} is by autophagy [134]. However, saturation of the autolysosomal degradation process can release PrP^{TSE} aggregates and degradation enzymes into the neuroplasm contributing to autophagy upregulation and neuronal death [134]. Nevertheless, although autophagy-inducing agents delayed disease onset and PrP^{TSE} accumulation in the CNS of mice [152], survival time was not modified [153]. Along this line, neither autophagy-inducing nor -inhibiting treatments altered the time course or amplitude of prion-induced neuronal death, strongly suggesting that autophagy in protein misfolding diseases is a secondary mechanism in the neurodegenerative process [141, 154].

3. Neuronal death in prion protein-deficient mice

3.1 Impaired autophagy in Zrch-1 prion protein-deficient mice

With the exception of the *Prnp*-knockout models in which ectopic expression of Doppel (Dpl) in the CNS leads to PC death, most other *Prnp*-knockout mouse models do not show gross abnormalities indicating that PrP^c may be dispensable for embryonic development and adulthood. Nevertheless, PrP-deficient mice exhibit an increased predilection for seizures, motor and cognitive disabilities, reduced synaptic inhibition, and long term potentiation in the hippocampus. Also, altered development of the granule cell layer, dysregulation of the cerebellar network and age-dependent spongiform changes with reactive astrogliosis have been observed [155, 156]. In cultures of PrP-deficient hippocampal neurons, autophagy is upregulated in the absence of serum or by hydrogen peroxide-induced oxidative stress [148, 157] suggesting that suppression of the protective effects of PrP^c could impair the autophagic flux in PrP-deficient neurons *in vivo*. Indeed, ultrastructural examination of hippocampus and cerebral cortex of ZH-I *Prnp*$^{0/0}$ mice revealed an accumulation of autophagosomes containing incompletely digested material increasing from 3 to 12 months of age [158]. In addition, an ultrastructural examination of PCs in the cerebellum of ZH-I *Prnp*$^{0/0}$ mice revealed significant autophagic accumulation in the somato-dendritic compartment of these neurons from 6 to 14.5 months of age (**Figure 11**). Since autophagic cell death is known to induce neurodegeneration [136, 159, 160], these signs of autophagy blockade could reflect a sustained, progressive autophagic neuronal loss in the CNS of the ZH-I *Prnp*$^{0/0}$ mice.

3.2 Neuronal loss in Dpl-expressing Ngsk prion protein-deficient mice

Nagasaki (Ngsk) PrP-deficient mice which have a deletion of the entire *Prnp* gene [161–163] develop progressive cerebellar ataxia, which was later discovered to result from the absence of a splice acceptor site in exon 3 of *Prnp* [164]. This leads to the aberrant overexpression of the *Prnd* gene encoding the PrP^c paralogue Dpl [165, 166] that causes selective degeneration of cerebellar PCs. Notably, the reintroduction of *Prnp* in mice overexpressing *Prnd* in the brain rescued the phenotype, suggesting a functional link between the two proteins [167]. Dpl has been shown to have intrinsic neurotoxic properties in cerebellar neurons [168] and has been proposed to interfere with PrP^c and affect cell survival [100]. According to this hypothesis, PrP^c and Dpl bind a common ligand LPrP, where PrP^c binding induces a cell survival signal while Dpl binding activates a death signaling cascade. In PrP^c-deficient *Prnp*-knockout mice that do not express Dpl, the existence of a protein

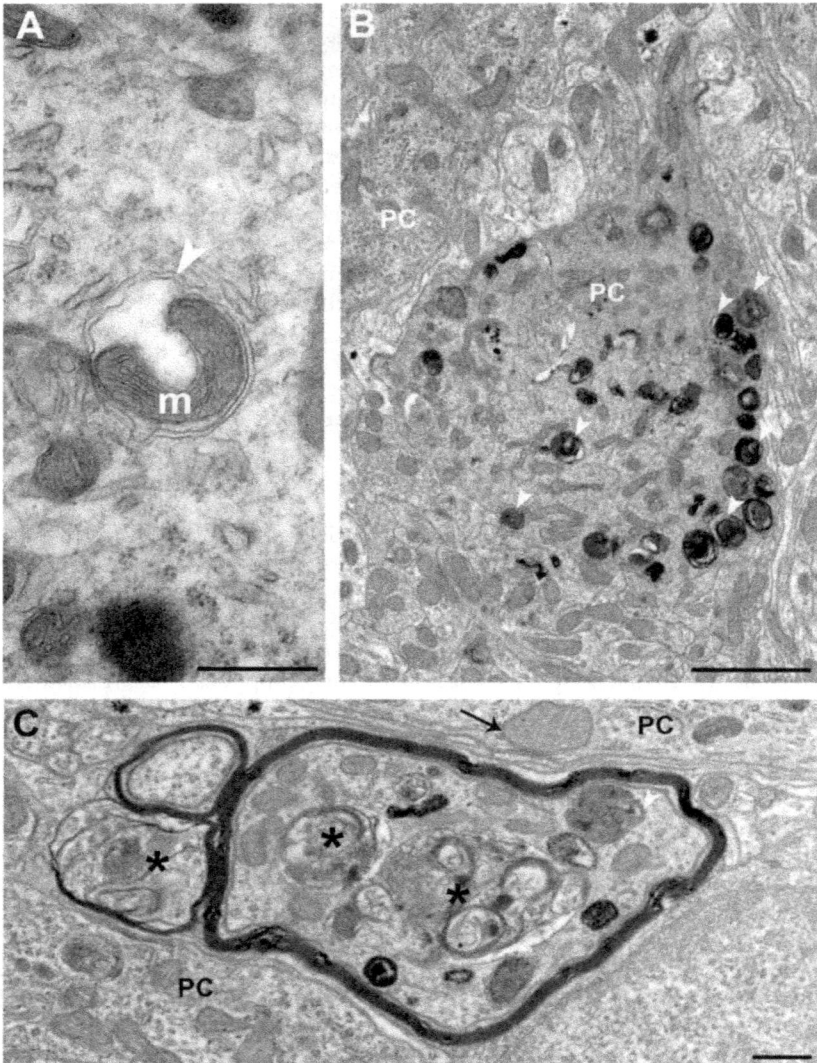

Figure 11.
Autophagy in ZH-I Prnp⁰/⁰ PCs. A. Mitophagy in the PC neuroplasm of a 4.5 months-old ZH-I Prnp⁰/⁰ mouse. Arrowhead shows the double membrane of an autophagic vacuole sequestrating a mitochondrion (m). Scale bar = 500 nm. B, C. 12 months-old ZH-I Prnp⁰/⁰ mice. PC layer. B. Autophagic PC containing numerous autophagosomes and autolysosomes (arrowheads). Scale bar = 2 μm. C. PC layer. Degenerating PC axons containing autophagosomes and lysosomes (*). Scale bar =500 nm.

π has been proposed to induce a cell survival signal when bound to LPrP [169]. For the moment, LPrP and π remain to be identified, as well as the neuronal death pathways involved in Dpl-induced PC loss.

Because Dpl neurotoxicity depends on PrP^c-deficiency in PCs, investigating the underlying neurotoxic mechanism may provide important insight into the neuroprotective function of PrP^c. The resistance of the PC population to neurotoxicity increased in the cerebellum of Ngsk mice, which were either deficient for the pro-apoptotic factor Bax [121] or over-express the anti-apoptotic factor Bcl-2 [170]. Although this suggests that an intrinsic apoptotic process is involved in the death of the Ngsk *Prnp⁰/⁰* PCs, a significant PC loss still occurred in both

(Bax$^{-/-}$; Ngsk $Prnp^{0/0}$) and (HuBcl-2; Ngsk $Prnp^{0/0}$) double mutants. Thus, the Ngsk condition, i.e., Dpl neurotoxicity and PrP-deficiency, could activate BAX-independent mechanisms in the Ngsk $Prnp^{0/0}$ PCs. These neurons exhibited robust autophagy well before significant neuronal death in the cerebellar cortex of the Ngsk $Prnp^{0/0}$ mice [135, 171] suggesting that either "reactive" autophagy is initially induced as a neuroprotective response to Dpl neurotoxicity or impaired autophagy results from PrP-deficiency as in ZH-I $Prnp^{0/0}$ mice (see above and [158]). Indeed, the increased expression of the autophagic markers SCRG1, LC3-II, and P62 proteins without any changes in mRNA levels, indicates that the ultimate steps of autophagic degradation are impaired in Ngsk $Prnp^{0/0}$ PCs [135]. Probably due to this impairment of autophagic proteolysis, LC3-II-, and Lamp-1-labeled autophagosomes and autolysosomes [172] accumulate in the Ngsk $Prnp^{0/0}$ PCs. How apoptosis and autophagy are involved in Ngsk $Prnp^{0/0}$ PC death remains to be determined.

To further investigate the role of autophagy in the death of Ngsk $Prnp^{0/0}$ PCs, a quantitative analysis of autophagic PCs was performed at the ultrastructural level in the cerebellum of Ngsk $Prnp^{0/0}$, Bax$^{-/-}$; Ngsk $Prnp^{0/0}$, ZCH-I $Prnp^{0/0}$ and control Bax$^{+/+}$;$Prnp^{+/+}$ mice (**Figure 12**). At 4.5 months of age, equivalent amounts of autophagic somato-dendritic compartments and axons of PCs were found in the cerebella of Ngsk $Prnp^{0/0}$ and Bax$^{-/-}$; Ngsk $Prnp^{0/0}$ mutants and were significantly more than those in ZCH-I $Prnp^{0/0}$ and control Bax$^{+/+}$;Prnp$^{+/+}$ cerebella. Interestingly, the amounts of autophagic axons and somato-dendritic compartments of PCs in the ZCH-I $Prnp^{0/0}$ and control Bax$^{+/+}$;$Prnp^{+/+}$ cerebella were not different. These data suggest that while autophagy induction is already visible in PCs with the Ngsk condition, it is not induced in control Bax$^{+/+}$;$Prnp^{+/+}$ PCs, nor in the absence of PrP^c in the ZCH-I $Prnp^{0/0}$ PCs. Thus, autophagy seems to be induced by Dpl neurotoxicity in the Ngsk condition whether BAX is present or not; whereas PrP-deficiency alone has no autophagy-inducing effect at this age (**Figure 13**).

At 6.5–7 months of age, the amount of autophagic somato-dendritic compartments and axons of PC were significantly decreased in Bax$^{-/-}$; Ngsk $Prnp^{0/0}$ cerebella compared with Ngsk $Prnp^{0/0}$ cerebella. Consequently, the amount of autophagic PC profiles in the Bax$^{-/-}$; Ngsk $Prnp^{0/0}$ and ZH-I $Prnp^{0/0}$ cerebella was equivalent, yet more than in the control Bax$^{+/+}$;$Prnp^{+/+}$ cerebella. Furthermore, autophagic PC somato-dendritic compartments and axons did not change from 4.5 to 6.5–7 months of age in the Bax$^{-/-}$; Ngsk $Prnp^{0/0}$, whereas many more PCs were autophagic in the 6.5–7 month-old compared to the 4.5 month-old Ngsk $Prnp^{0/0}$ cerebella. This increase was also observed in ZH-I $Prnp^{0/0}$ cerebella, while no autophagic PCs were found in 6.5–7 month-old control Bax$^{+/+}$;$Prnp^{+/+}$ cerebella (**Figure 13**).

This suggests that BAX-deficiency modulates autophagy in Ngsk $Prnp^{0/0}$ PCs after 4.5 months of age. Autophagy in the ZH-I $Prnp^{0/0}$ PCs had increased to the same level as observed in the Bax$^{-/-}$;Ngsk $Prnp^{0/0}$ cerebella. Thus, the persistent autophagy in the PCs of the Bax$^{-/-}$;Ngsk $Prnp^{0/0}$ double mutants is likely related to PrP-deficiency. Also, autophagy- and Bax-dependent apoptosis are likely to occur in the same PCs that are rescued by Bax deletion.

At 12 months of age, the amount of autophagic somato-dendritic compartments and axons of PCs in Bax$^{-/-}$;Ngsk $Prnp^{0/0}$ cerebella was equivalent to that found in 4.5 month-old cerebella suggesting that autophagy remains stable in this PC population, at a level similar to that maintained in the ZH-I $Prnp^{0/0}$, and this likely results from PrP-deficiency. Indeed, many more autophagic PC somato-dendritic compartments and axons were observed in ZH-I $Prnp^{0/0}$ cerebella than in the cerebella of 12 month-old control Bax$^{+/+}$;$Prnp^{+/+}$ mice which did not contain autophagic PCs. However, the autophagic PC somato-dendritic compartments were

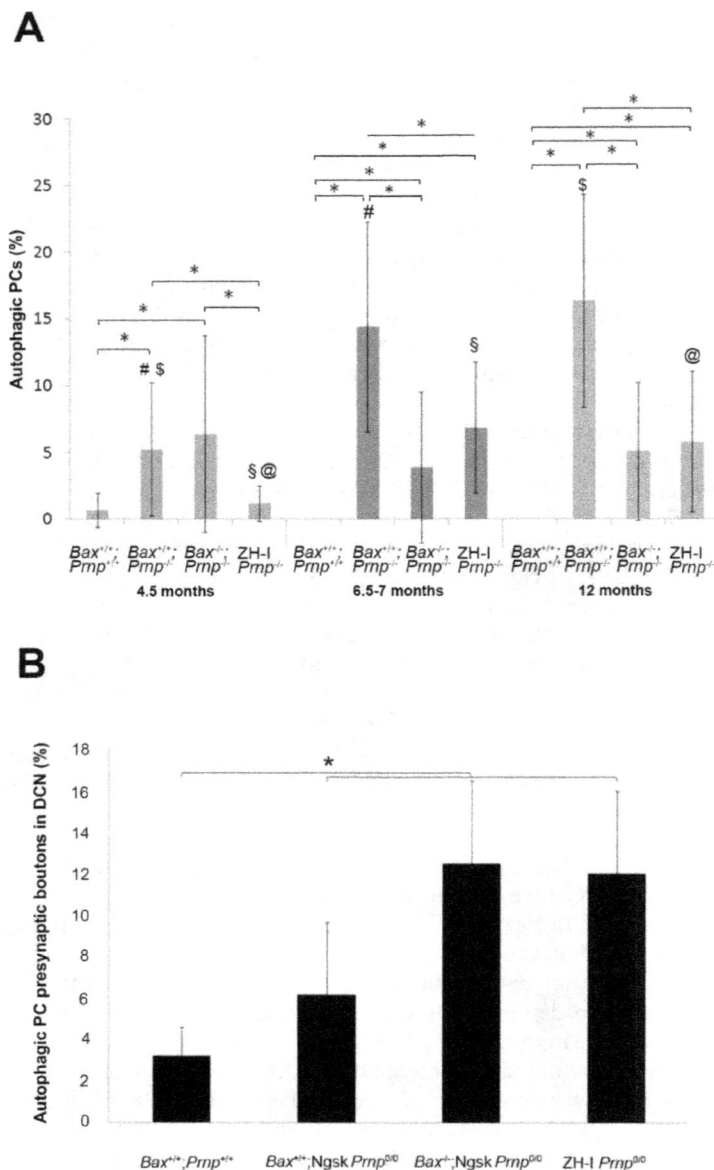

Figure 12.
Quantitative analysis of autophagy in PCs of control Bax$^{+/+}$;Prnp$^{+/+}$ and PrP-deficient Bax$^{+/+}$;Ngsk Prnp$^{o/o}$, Bax$^{-/-}$;Ngsk Prnp$^{o/o}$ and ZH-I Prnp$^{o/o}$ mutant mice. Autophagic somato-dendritic and axonal profiles were counted in 200 PCs in transverse cerebellar sections (50 PCs per hemisphere and hemivermis) from each mouse at 4.5, 6.5–7 and 12 months of age (n = 3 mice/age/genotype). PC soma, primary dendrite and axons were autophagic when containing three or more autophagic profiles (phagophore, autophagosome, autophagolysosome). Data are given as mean values ± standard deviation (SD). Statistical comparisons between ages and genotypes were performed using a two-tailed Student's t test (Statistica). A. Mean percentages of autophagic PC somato-dendritic and axonal compartments. *, #, @, \$, §: p < 0.01. B. Mean percentages of autophagic PC presynaptic boutons making symmetrical synapses on somato-dendritic profiles of deep cerebellar neurons. The PC presynaptic boutons were autophagic when containing at least one autophagic organelle. Autophagic PC presynaptic boutons were counted in 300 presynaptic boutons selected randomly in either left or right fastigial, interposed and dentate nuclei (100 boutons/nucleus) in three 12 month-old mice of each genotype. Statistical comparisons between genotypes were performed using a two-tailed Student's t test (Statistica) and given as mean values ± standard deviation (SD). *, p < 0.01.

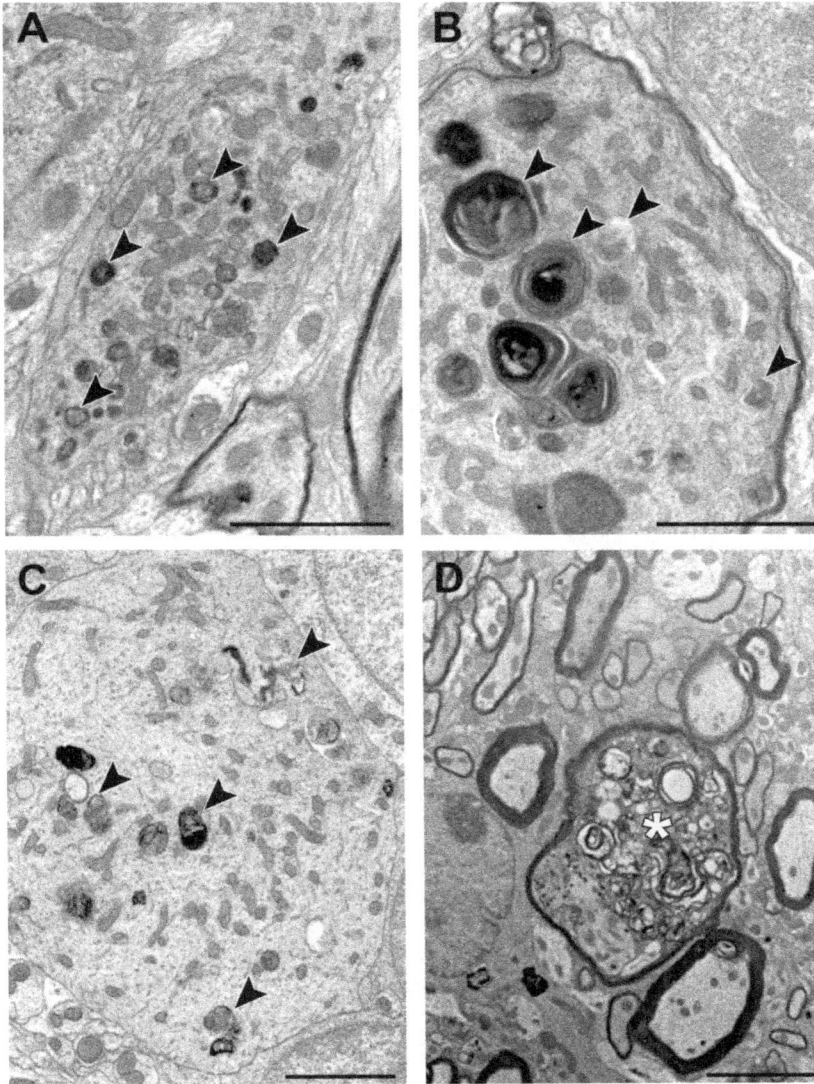

Figure 13.
*Autophagy in PCs of 7 (A, B) and 12 (C, D) month-old Bax$^{-/-}$;Ngsk Prnp$^{0/0}$ mice. **A**. PC-like somato-dendritic profile containing numerous autophagic vacuoles and autolysosomes (arrowheads) in the PC layer. **B**. Autolysosomes (arrowheads) in a dystrophic PC-like, myelinated axonal profile in the internal granular layer. **C**. Autophagic vacuoles and autolysosomes in a PC-like somato-dendritic profile. **D**. Autophagic PC-like myelinated axon (*). Scale bars = 2 μm.*

still more in Ngsk $Prnp^{0/0}$ cerebella (16.36 ± 7.9) compared with $Bax^{-/-}$;Ngsk $Prnp^{0/0}$ (5.08 ± 5) cerebella, and there was a significant increase from 6.5–7 (14.38 ± 7.8) to 12 months of age. The increased amount of autophagic PC axons in $Bax^{-/-}$;Ngsk $Prnp^{0/0}$ cerebella was stable during this same period (3.9 ± 5.6 at 6.5–7 months; 5.08 ± 5.1 at 12 months), suggesting that the initiation of axonal autophagy peaks at 6.5–7 months of age (**Figure 12**) [135, 171, 173–176]. In agreement, an examination of autophagy in the presynaptic terminals of PCs impinging on the somato-dendritic compartments of the deep nuclear neurons in the fastigial, interposed and dentate

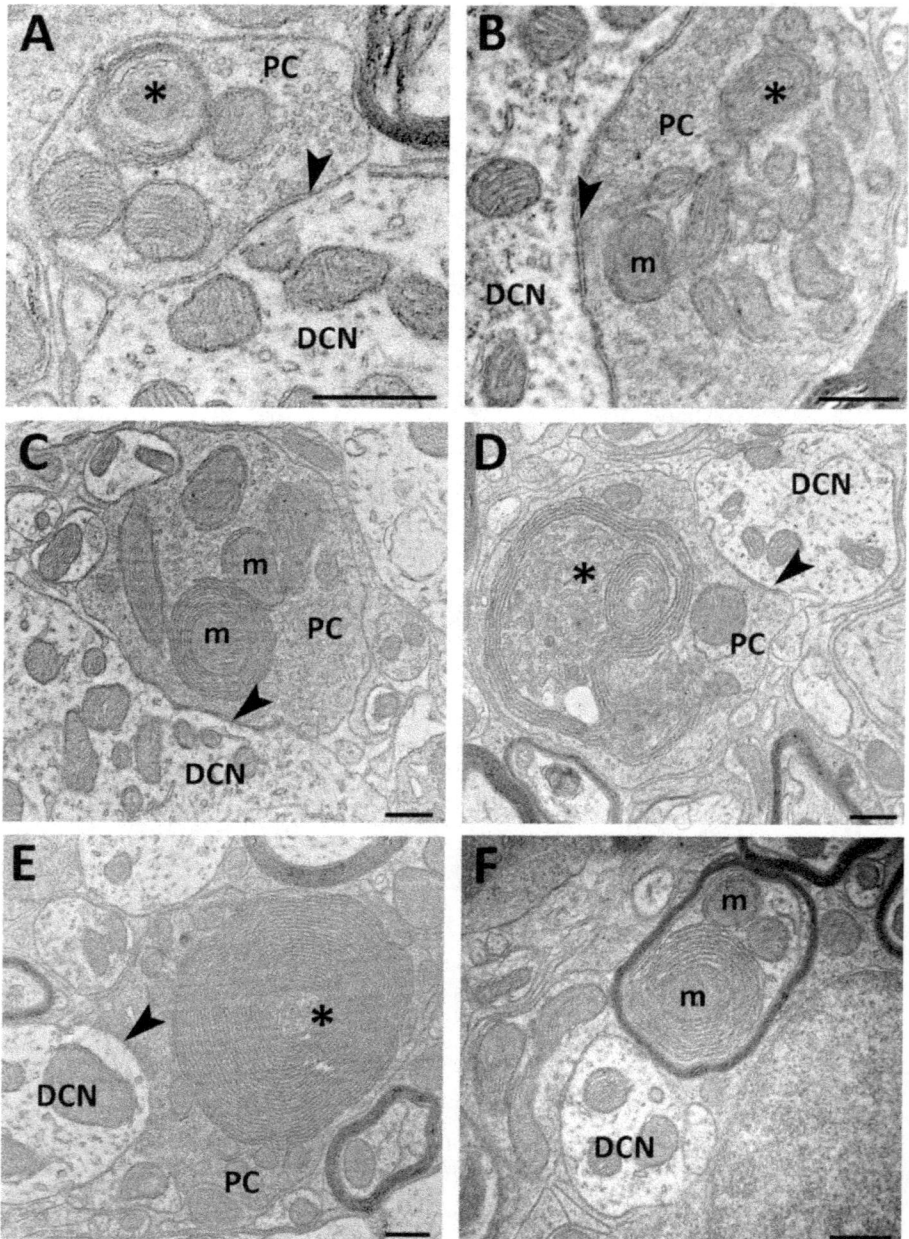

Figure 14.
*Autophagy in the deep cerebellar nuclei of 13 month-old Ngsk (A, C–F) and 10 month-old ZH-I (B) Prnp°/°
mice. A–E. PC presynaptic boutons establishing symmetrical synapses (arrowheads) with somato-dendritic
profiles of deep cerebellar neurons (DCN) and containing different stages of double-membrane wraps
sequestrating neuroplasm (* in A, B, D, E) and mitochondria (m in C, F). F. Myelinated PC-like axon with
mitophagic profiles. Scale bars = 500 nm.*

deep cerebellar nuclei, revealed a significantly greater amount of autophagic
PC presynaptic boutons in the deep nuclei of all mutants compared to control
$Bax^{+/+};Prnp^{+/+}$ mice (**Figure 14**).

The absence of BAX not only protected some PCs from neurotoxicity in the cerebellum of the Ngsk $Prnp^{0/0}$ mice [121], but also decreased the number of autophagic neurons suggesting that the PCs rescued by *Bax* deficiency do not display activated autophagy, whereas the autophagic PCs in the $Bax^{-/-}$;Ngsk $Prnp^{0/0}$ cerebellum are likely to result from PrP-deficiency as in the ZH-I $Prnp^{0/0}$ cerebellum. Nevertheless, the persistent loss of $Bax^{-/-}$;Ngsk $Prnp^{0/0}$ PCs could result from an increased sensitivity of these PCs to the Ngsk condition compared to ZH-I $Prnp^{0/0}$ PCs.

The complex pattern of neuronal death observed in neurodegenerative diseases is believed to involve an extensive interplay between the major cell death pathways [177, 178]. This is likely the case in prion-infected, as well as PrP-deficient neurons such as PCs. We further investigated PC death in Ngsk $Prnp^{0/0}$ and ZH-I $Prnp^{0/0}$ COCS by measuring PC survival and development using morphometric methods [179] in COCS from these PrP-deficient mice. Similar timing and amplitude of PC growth impairment and death were observed in all PrP-deficient genotypes. Indeed, PC surface, perimeter, and dendritic extension increased between 7 and 21 DIV in the wild-type COCS, while no significant variation of surface and perimeter could be measured in the PrP-deficient mutant COCS during this period (**Figure 15**). Similarly, wild-type and PrP-deficient PCs displayed equivalent maximal dendritic extension after 7 days *ex vivo*, but wild-type PCs continued to increase their maximal dendritic length until 21 DIV, while the dendrites of PrP-deficient PCs did not grow during this period [14, 180]. Thus, PrP-deficient PCs exhibit a similar developmental deficit which seems to be independent of Dpl expression in COCS.

The neurotoxic effects of PrP-deficiency were quantitatively analyzed by counting PCs at 3, 5, 7, 12, and 21 days in COCS from wild-type, Ngsk $Prnp^{+/0}$, Ngsk $Prnp^{0/0}$, and ZH-I $Prnp^{0/0}$. Whereas, wild-type PCs' numbers remained stable during the whole period, severe PC loss (68–69%) had occurred at 7 DIV and slightly increased up to 21 DIV in all PrP-deficient mutant COCS. PC loss displayed similar kinetics and amplitude in Ngsk $Prnp^{+/0}$, Ngsk $Prnp^{0/0}$, and ZH-I $Prnp^{0/0}$ COCS suggesting that despite detectable levels of 15–20 kDa glycosylated form of Dpl in the Ngsk $Prnp^{0/0}$ COCS (**Figure 16**), it may be not implicated in PC death in *ex vivo* cultures.

Furthermore, at the ultrastructural level, whereas autophagic organelles were rare in wild-type PCs after 7 and 12 DIV, Ngsk $Prnp^{0/0}$ PCs contained numerous autophagosomes and autophagolysosomes at different maturation stages (**Figure 17**). During the period of PC death in the $Prnp^{0/0}$ COCS (i.e., 3, 5, and 7 DIV) Western blotting of apoptotic and autophagic markers revealed a 4- to 5-fold increase in markers of autophagosomal formation such as LC3B-II (at 5 DIV), p62, and beclin-1 (at 3 and 5 DIV) in the ZH-I and Ngsk $Prnp^{0/0}$ COCS and the lysosomal receptor LAMP-1 in the Ngsk $Prnp^{0/0}$ COCS at 7 DIV (**Figure 18**). Increased amounts of activated caspase-3 indicated the apoptosis in protein extracts of COCS from both $Prnp^{0/0}$ genotypes as early as 3DIV [14].

This morphometric and quantitative analysis of COCS suggests that PrP-deficiency, rather than Dpl neurotoxicity, is responsible for the neuronal growth deficit and loss *ex vivo*. Indeed, the neurotoxic properties of Dpl did not seem to contribute to Ngsk PC loss in the COCS, whereas Dpl-induced PC loss is detectable in 6-month-old Ngsk $Prnp^{0/0}$ mice. A possible explanation for this difference is that COCS are not mature enough to model 6-month-old cerebellar tissue. Nevertheless, in Ngsk $Prnp^{0/0}$ and ZH-I $Prnp^{0/0}$ COCs, activation of autophagy and apoptosis is contemporaneous with the atrophy and death of PCs during the first week of culture suggesting that PrP-deficiency is solely responsible for neuronal death in this

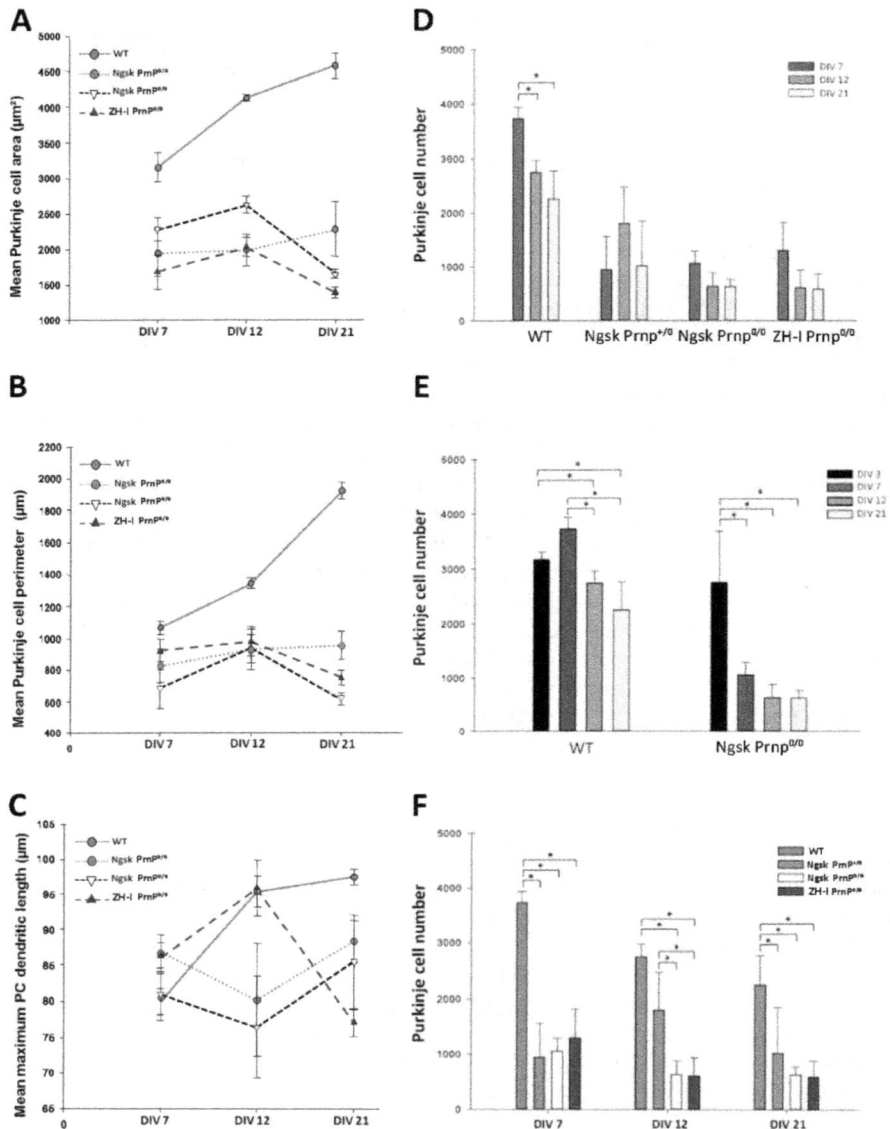

Figure 15.
*PC growth deficits and loss in PrP-deficient COCS. **A, B**. PC area (A) and perimeter (B) of WT PCs increased from DIV7 to DIV21, whereas both dimensions in Ngsk Prnp$^{+/0}$, Ngsk Prnp$^{0/0}$ and ZH-I Prnp$^{0/0}$ PCs did not change during the same period. A. At DIV7, WT PC area was larger than area of PrP-deficient PCs. **C**. While the longest dendrite of WT PCs had significantly grown from DIV7 to DIV21, the longest dendrite of PrP-deficient PCs displayed similar growth impairment suggesting that in both Ngsk and ZH-I conditions, PrP-deficiency is responsible for PC growth deficits. **D–F**. PC loss occurred progressively during the DIV7-DIV21 period in WT COCS (40% at DIV21) while similar loss of PrP-deficient PCs had occurred in the Ngsk Prnp$^{+/0}$, Ngsk Prnp$^{0/0}$ (40%) and ZH-I Prnp$^{0/0}$ (55%) COCS as early as DIV7. **E**. The Ngsk Prnp$^{0/0}$ COCS had lost many more PCs than the WT COCS over the DIV3-DIV7 period indicating a neurotoxic effect during this period that is attributable to PrP-deficiency since the Ngsk and the ZH-I conditions induced similar neuronal loss at DIV7.*

ex vivo system and that PrP^{c} is neuroprotective for cerebellar PCs. As ZH-I *Prnp*$^{0/0}$ PCs survive *in vivo*, PC death in ZH-I *Prnp*$^{0/0}$ and Ngsk *Prnp*$^{0/0}$ COCS could result from a noxious exacerbation of PrP-deficiency by *ex vivo* conditions.

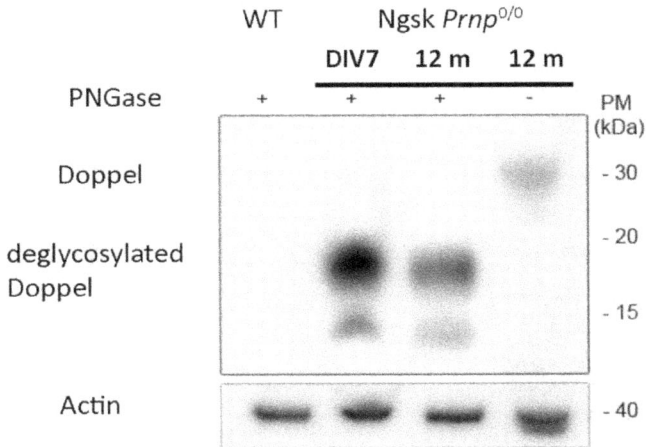

Figure 16.
Western blot of Dpl in Ngsk Prnp^{o/o} DIV7 COCS and 12 month-old mouse cerebellum. Dpl was detected in a Ngsk Prnp^{o/o} COCS at DIV7 and in situ in the cerebellar extract from a 12 month-old Ngsk Prnp^{o/o} mouse but not in the cerebellum of a wild-type (WT) mouse. Dpl migrates at 15–20 kDa after deglycosylation by peptide N-glucosidase (PNGase).

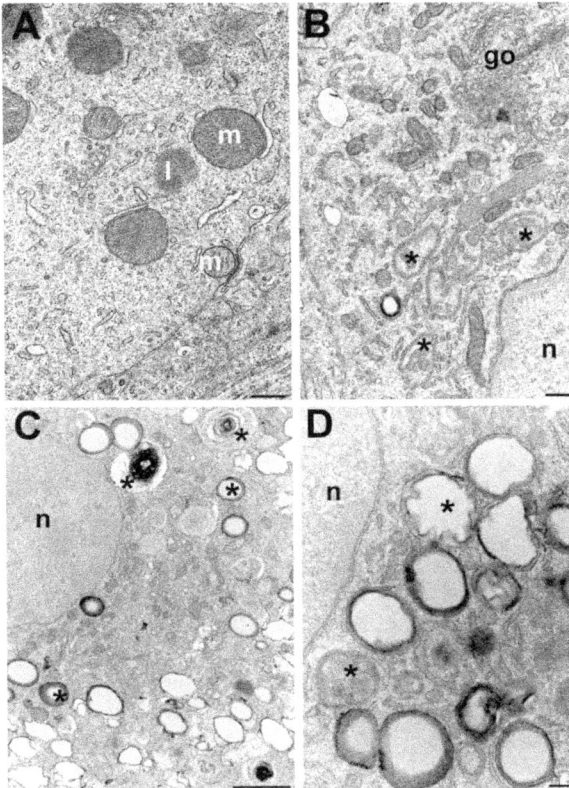

Figure 17.
*Autophagy in Ngsk Prnp^{o/o} PCs ex vivo. **A**. PC cytoplasm in a 12 DIV WT COCS. m, mitochondrion; l, lysosome. Scale bar = 500 nm. **B–D**. Autophagic PC cytoplasm in 7 DIV Ngsk Prnp^{o/o} COCSs. Asterisks indicate nascent autophagic vacuoles in B and different maturation stages of autophagolysosomes in C and D. n, nucleus. Scale bar = 2 μm.*

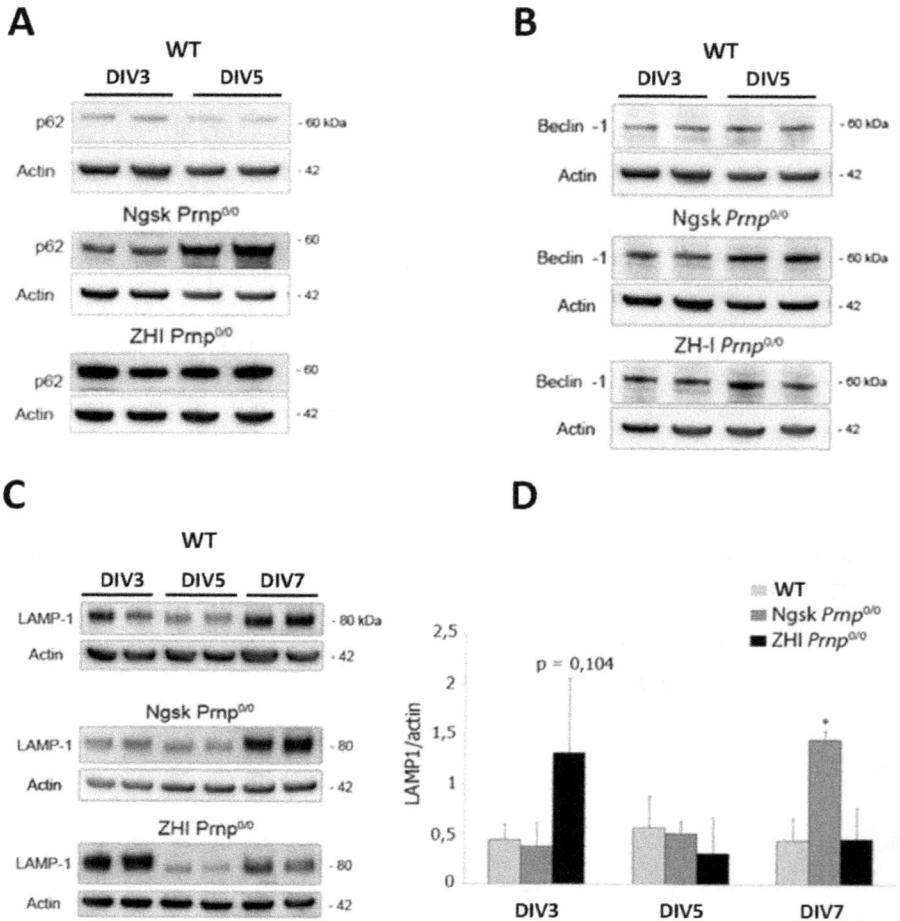

Figure 18.
*Western blot of autophagic markers p62, beclin-1 and LAMP-1. **A**. p62 and **B**. Beclin-1. The markers were weakly expressed in WT COCS, but increased in DIV3 and DIV5 COCS from PrP-deficient mice. **C, D**. LAMP-1 did not vary in WT and ZH-1 COCS from DIV3 to DIV7, but increased in DIV7 Ngsk Prnp$^{0/0}$ COCS indicating increased lysosomal activity (p < 0.05; n = 3 mice/genotype and DIV).*

4. Conclusion

Although the contribution of apoptosis to prion-induced death of central neurons including cerebellar ones is strongly supported, our studies of scrapie-infected PCs show that although caspase-3 is activated, the pro-apoptotic BAX/BCL-2-dependent mitochondrial pathway is not involved in the prion-induced death of these neurons. This is also the case for BSE-induced death of hippocampal and thalamic neurons [119], suggesting that prions exert neurotoxicity through BAX-independent activation of caspase-3. Ultrastructural evidence of ER stress and robust autophagy in the scrapie-infected cerebellar neurons both *in vivo* and *ex vivo* implicate them in these BAX-independent neurotoxic mechanisms. Furthermore, the autophagic blockade resulting from prion protein-deficiency in ZH-I and Ngsk *Prnp$^{0/0}$* mice may contribute to neuronal death in infectious prion-diseased cerebellar neurons. In Ngsk *Prnp$^{0/0}$* cerebellar neurons, Dpl neurotoxicity and PrP-deficiency contribute to neuronal death probably through an interplay between autophagic blockade and BAX-dependent apoptosis.

Author details

Audrey Ragagnin[1], Qili Wang[1], Aurélie Guillemain[1], Siaka Dole[1],
Anne-Sophie Wilding[1], Valérie Demais[1,2], Cathy Royer[1,2], Anne-Marie Haeberlé[1],
Nicolas Vitale[1], Stéphane Gasman[1], Nancy Grant[1] and Yannick Bailly[1*]

1 Intracellular Membrane Trafficking in the Nervous and Neuroendocrine System,
INCI, CNRS UPR3212, University of Strasbourg, Strasbourg, France

2 In Vitro Imaging Platform, CNRS UPS 3156, University of Strasbourg, Strasbourg,
France

*Address all correspondence to: byan@inci-cnrs.unistra.fr

IntechOpen

References

[1] Collinge J. Prion diseases of human and animals: Their causes and molecular basis. Annual Review of Neuroscience. 2001;**24**:519-550

[2] Morales R. Prion strains in mammals: Different conformations leading to disease. PLoS Pathogens. 2017;**13**:e1006323. DOI: 10.1371/journal.ppat.1006323

[3] Ironside JW, Ritchie DL. Head MW prion diseases. Handbook of Clinical Neurology. 2018;**145**:393-403. DOI: 10.1016/B978-0-12-802395-2.00028-6

[4] Babelhadj B, Di Bari MA, Pirisinu L, Chiappini B, Gaouar SBS, Riccardi G, et al. Prion disease in dromedary camels, Algeria. Emerging Infectious Diseases. Jun 2018;**24**(6):1029-1036. DOI: 10.3201/eid2406.172007

[5] Prusiner S. Novel proteinaceous infection particles cause scrapie. Science. 1982;**216**:136-144

[6] Brandner S, Raeber A, Sailer A, Blättler T, Fischer M, Weissmann C, et al. Normal host prion protein (PrPC) is required for scrapie spread within the central nervous system. Proceedings of the National Academy of Sciences of the United States of America. 1996;**93**:13148-13151

[7] Aguzzi A, Polymenidou M. Mammalian prion biology: One century of evolving concepts. Cell. 2004;**116**:313-327

[8] Büeler HR, Fischer M, Lang Y, Bluethmann H, Lipp HP, DeArmond SJ, et al. Normal development and behaviour of mice lacking the neuronal cell-surface PrP protein. Nature. 1992;**356**:577-582. DOI.org/10.1038/356577a0

[9] Manson JC, Clarke AR, Hooper ML, Aitchison L, McConnell I, Hope J. 129/Ola mice carrying a null mutation in PrP that abolishes mRNA production are developmentally normal. Molecular Neurobiology. 1994;**8**:121-127

[10] Nuvolone M, Hermann M, Scorce S, Russo G, Tiberi C, Schwarz P, et al. Strictly co-isogenic C57BL/6J-*Prnp*$^{-/-}$ mice: A rigorous resource for prion science. The Journal of Experimental Medicine. 2016;**213**:313-327

[11] Büeler H, Aguzzi A, Sailer A, Greiner RA, Autenried P, Aguet M, et al. Mice devoid of PrP are resistant to scrapie. Cell. 1993;**73**:1339-1347

[12] Mallucci GR, Ratte S, Asante EA, Linehan J, Gowland I, Jefferys JGR, et al. Post-natal knockout of prion protein alters hippocampal CA1 properties but does not result in neurodegeneration. The EMBO Journal. 2002;**21**:202-210

[13] Wulf MA, Senatore A, Aguzzi A. The biological function of the cellular prion protein: An update. BMC Biology. 2017;**15**:34. DOI: 10.1186/s12915-017-0375-5

[14] Ragagnin A, Guillemain A, Grant NJ, Bailly Y. Neuronal autophagy and prion proteins. In: Bailly YJR, editor. Autophagy—A Double-Edged Sword—Cell Survival or Death? Rijeka, Croatia: InTech Publisher; 2013. pp. 377-419

[15] Legname G. Elucidating the function of the prion protein. PLoS Pathogens. Aug 31, 2017;**13**(8):e1006458. DOI: 10.1371/journal.ppat.1006458

[16] Saa P, Harris D, Cervenakova L. Mechanisms of prion-induced neurodegeneration. Expert Reviews in Molecular Medicine. Apr 8, 2016;**18**:e5. DOI: 10.1017/erm2016.8

[17] Stahl N, Borchelt DR, Hsiao K, Prusiner SB. Scrapie prion protein

contain a phosphatidylinositol glycolipid. Cell. 1987;**51**:229-240

[18] Lainé J, Marc M, Sy M, Axelrad H. Cellular and subcellular morphological localization of normal prion protein in rodent cerebellum. The European Journal of Neuroscience. 2001;**14**:47-56

[19] Bailly Y, Haeberlé AM, Blanquet-Grossard F, Chasserot-Golaz S, Grant N, Schulze T, et al. Prion protein (PrP^c) immunocytochemistry and expression of the green fluorescent protein reporter gene under the control of bovine PrP gene promoter in the mouse brain. The Journal of Comparative Neurology. 2004;**473**:244-269

[20] Jacobson K, Dietrich C. Looking at lipid rafts? Trends in Cell Biology. 1999;**9**:87-91

[21] Mouillet-Richard S, Ermonval M, Chebassier C, Laplanche JL, Lehmann S, Launay JM, et al. Signal transduction through prion protein. Science. 2000;**289**:1925-1928. Epub Sep 16, 2000. DOI: 10.1126/science.289.5486.1925

[22] Linden R, Martins VR, Prado MA, Cammarota M, Izquierdo I, Brentani RR. Physiology of the prion protein. Physiological Reviews. 2008;**88**:673-728

[23] Bendheim PE, Brown HR, Rudelli RD, Scala LJ, Goller NL, Wen GY, et al. Nearly ubiquitous tissue distribution of the scrapie agent precursor protein. Neurology. 1992;**42**:149

[24] Haeberlé AM, Ribaut-Barassin C, Bombarde G, Mariani J, Hunsmann G, Grassi J, et al. Synaptic prion protein immuno-reactivity in the rodent cerebellum. Microscopy Research and Technique. 2000;**50**:66-75

[25] Salès N, Rodolfo K, Hässig R, Faucheux B, Di Giamberardino L, Moya KL. Cellular prion protein localization in rodent and primate brain. The European Journal of Neuroscience. 1998;**10**:2464-2471

[26] Salès N, Hässig R, Rodolfo K, Di Giamberardino L, Traiffort E, Ruat M, et al. Developmental expression of the cellular prion protein in elongating axons. The European Journal of Neuroscience. 2002;**15**:1163-1177

[27] Fournier JG, Escaig-Haye F, Billette de Villemeur T, Robain O. Ultrastructural localization of cellular prion protein (PrPc)in synaptic boutons of normal hamster hippocampus. Comptes Rendus de l'Académie des Sciences, Paris. 1995;**318**:339-344

[28] Herms J, Tings T, Gall S, Madlung A, Giese A, Siebert H, et al. Evidence of presynaptic location and function of the prion protein. The Journal of Neuroscience. 1999;**19**:8866-8875

[29] Mironov A, Latawiec D, Wille H, Bouzamondo-Bernstein E, Legname G, Williamson RA, et al. Cytosolic prion protein in neurons. The Journal of Neuroscience. 2003;**23**:183-193

[30] Borchelt DR, Koliatsos VE, Guarnieri M, Pardo CA, Sisodia SS, Price DL. Rapid anterograde axonal transport of the cellular prion glycoprotein in the peripheral and central nervous systems. The Journal of Biological Chemistry. 1994;**269**:14711-14714

[31] Moya K, Hässig R, Créminon C, Laffont I, Di Giamberardino L. Enhanced detection and retrograde axonal transport of PrPc in peripheral nerve. Journal of Neurochemistry. 2003;**88**:155-160

[32] Jeffrey M, Halliday WG, Bell J, Johnston AR, McLeod NK, Ingham C, et al. Synapse loss associated with abnormal PrP precedes neuronal degeneration

in the scrapie-infected murine hippocampus. Neuropathology and Applied Neurobiology. 2000;**26**:41-54

[33] Siskova Z, Reynolds RA, O'Connor V, Perry VH. Brain region specific presynaptic and postsynaptic degeneration are early components of neuropathology in prion diseases. PLoS One. 2013;**8**(1):e55004. DOI: 110.1371/journal.pone.0055004

[34] Senatore A, Colleoni S, Verderio C, Restelli E, Morini R, Condliffe SB, et al. Mutant PrP suppresses glutamatergic neurotransmission in cerebellar granule neurons by impairing membrane delivery of VGCC α2δ-1 subunit. Neuron. 2012;**74**:300-313. DOI: 10.1016/j.neuron.2012.02.027

[35] Khosravani H, Zhang Y, Tsutsui S, Hameed S, Altier C, Hamid J, et al. Prion protein attenuates excitotoxicity by inhibiting NMDA receptors. The Journal of Cell Biology. 2008;**181**:551-565. DOI: 10.1083/jcb.200711002

[36] Mercer RCC, Ma L, Watts JC, Strome R, Wohlgemuth S, Yang J, et al. The prion protein modulates A-typeK+ currents mediated by Kv4.2 complexes through dipeptidyl aminopeptidase-like protein 6. The Journal of Biological Chemistry. 2013;**288**:37241-37255

[37] Stys PK, You H, Zamponi GW. Copper-dependent regulation of NMDA receptors by cellular prion protein: Implications for neurodegenerative disorders. The Journal of Physiology. 2012;**590**:1357-1368. DOI: 10.1113/jphysiol.2011.225276

[38] Gasperini L, Meneghette E, Pastore B, Benetti F, Legname G. Prion protein and copper cooperatively protect neurons by modulating NMDA receptors through S-nitrosylation. Antioxidants & Redox Signaling. 2015;**22**:772-784

[39] Muller WE, Ushijima H, Schroder HC, Forrest JM, Schatton WF, Rytik PG, et al. Cytoprotective effect of NMDA receptor antagonists on prion protein (PrioSc)-induced toxicity in rat cortical cell cultures. European Journal of Pharmacology. 1993;**246**:261-267

[40] Resenberger UK, Harmeier A, Woerner AC, Goodman JL, Muller V, Krishnan R, et al. The cellular prion protein mediates neurotoxic signalling of eIF2α-sheet-rich conformers independent of prion replication. The EMBO Journal. 2011;**30**:2057-2070. DOI: 10.1038/emboj.2011.86

[41] Carulla P, Llorens F, Matamoros-Angles A, Aguilar-Calvo P, Espinosa JC, Gavín R, et al. Involvement of PrP(C) in kainate-induced excitotoxicity in several mouse strains. Scientific Reports. 2015;**5**:11971. DOI: 10.1038/srep11971

[42] Kleene R, Loers G, Langer J, Frobert Y, Buck F, Schachner M. Prion protein regulates glutamate-dependent lactate transport of astrocytes. The Journal of Neuroscience. 2007;**27**:12331-12340

[43] Watt NT, Taylor DR, Kerrigan TL, Griffiths HH, Rushworth JV, Whitehouse IJ, et al. Prion protein facilitates uptake of zinc into neuronal cells. Nature Communications. 2012;**3**:1134

[44] Beraldo FH, Arantes CP, Santos TG, Machado CF, Roffe M, Hajj GN, et al. Metabotropic glutamate receptors transducer signals for neurite outgrowth after binding of the prion protein to laminin γ1 chain. The FASEB Journal. 2011;**25**:265-279

[45] Um JW, Kaufman AC, Kostylev M, Heiss JK, Stagi M, Takahashi H, et al. Metabotropic glutamate receptor 5 is a coreceptor for Alzheimer eIF2α oligomer bound to cellular prion protein. Neuron. 2013;**79**:887-902

[46] Lauren J, Gimbel DA, Nygaard HB, Gilbert JW, Strittmatter SM. Cellular prion protein mediates impairment of synaptic plasticity by amyloid-β oligomers. Nature. 2009;**457**:1128-1132

[47] Um JW, Nygaard HB, Heiss JK, Kostylev MA, Stagi M, Wortmeyer A, et al. Alzheimer amyloid-β oligomer bound to postsynaptic prion protein activates Fyn to impair neurons. Nature Neuroscience. 2012;**15**:1227-1235

[48] Winklhofer KF, Tatzelt J, Haass C. The two faces of protein misfolding: Gain- and loss-of-function in neurodegenerative diseases. The EMBO Journal. 2008;**27**:336-349

[49] Harris DA, True HL. New insights into prion structure and toxicity. Neuron. 2006;**50**:353-357

[50] Moreno JA, Radford H, Peretti D, Steinert JR, Verity N, Martin MG, et al. Sustained translational repression by eIF2α-P mediates prion neurodegeneration Nature. 2012;**485**:507-511. DOI: 10.1038/nature11058. Erratum in: Nature. 2014;**511**:370

[51] McKinnon C, Goold R, Andre R, Devoy A, Ortega Z, Moonga J, et al. Prion-mediated neurodegeneration is associated with early impairment of the ubiquitin-proteasome system. Acta Neuropathologica. 2016;**131**:411-425. DOI: 10.1007/s00401-015-1508-y

[52] Hegde RS, Tremblay P, Groth D, DeArmond SJ, Prusiner SB, Lingappa VR. Transmissible and genetic prion diseases share a common pathway of neurodegeneration. Nature. 1999;**402**:822-826

[53] Moreno JA, Halliday M, Molloy C, Radford H, Verity N, Axten JM, et al. Oral treatment targeting the unfolded protein response prevents neurodegeneration and clinical

disease in prion-infected mice. Science Translational Medicine. Oct 9, 2013;**5**(206):206ra138. DOI: 10.1126/scitranslmed.3006767

[54] Telling GC. The importance of prions. PLoS Pathogens. 2013;**9**:e1003090. DOI: 10.1371/journal. ppat.1003090

[55] Piétri M, Dakowski C, Hannaoui S, Alleaume-Buteaux A, Hernandez-Rapp J, Ragagnin A, et al. PDK1 decreases TACE-mediated α-secretase activity and promotes disease progression in prion and Alzheimer's diseases. Nature Medicine. 2013;**19**:1124-1131

[56] Alleaume-Buteaux A, Nicot S, Piétri M, Baudry A, Dakowski C, Tixador P, et al. Double-edge sword of sustained ROCK activation in prion diseases through neuritogenesis defects and prion accumulation. PLoS Pathogens. 2015;**11**:e1005073

[57] Ezpeleta J, Boudet-Devaud F, Piétri M, Baudry A, Baudouin V, Alleaume-Buteaux A, et al. Protective role of cellular prion protein against TNFα-mediated inflammation through TACE α-secretase. Scientific Reports. 2017;**7**:7671. DOI: 10.1038/s41598-017-08110-x

[58] Hilton KJ, Cunningham C, Reynolds RA, Perry VH. Early hippocampal synaptic loss precedes neuronal loss and associates with early behavioural deficits in three distinct strains of prion disease. PLoS One. 2013;**8**:e68062. DOI: 10.1371/journal. pone.0068062

[59] Ragagnin A, Ezpeleta J, Guillemain A, Boudet-Devaud F, Haeberlé A-M, Demais V, et al. Cerebellar compartmentation of prion pathogenesis. Brain Pathology. 2017;**28**:240-263. DOI: 10.1111/bpa.12503

[60] Kristiansen M, Deriziotis P, Dimcheff DE, Jackson GS, Ovaa H, Naumann H, et al. Disease-associated prion protein oligomers inhibit the 26S proteasome. Molecular Cell. 2007;**26**:175-188

[61] Pietri M, Caprini A, Mouillet-Richard S, Pradines E, Ermonval M, Grassi J, et al. Overstimulation of PrPC signaling pathways by prion peptide 106-126 causes oxidative injury of bioaminergic neuronal cells. The Journal of Biological Chemistry. 2006;**281**:28470-28479

[62] Heiseke A, Aguib Y, Schatzl HM. Autophagy, prion infection and their mutual interactions. Current Issues in Molecular Biology. 2010;**12**:87-98

[63] Sikorska B. Mechanisms of neuronal death in transmissible spongiform encephalopathies. Folia Neuropathologica. 2004;**42**(Suppl B): 89-95

[64] Liberski PP, Brown DR, Sikorska B, Caughey B, Brown P. Cell death and autophagy in prion diseases (transmissible spongiform encephalopathies). Folia Neuropathologica. 2008;**46**:1-25

[65] Sikorska B, Liberski PP, Giraud P, Kopp N, Brown P. Autophagy is a part of ultrastructural synaptic pathology in Creutzfeldt-Jakob disease: A brain biopsy study. The International Journal of Biochemistry & Cell Biology. 2004;**36**:2563-2573

[66] Bruce ME, McBride PA, Jeffrey M, Scott JR. PrP in pathology and pathogenesis in scrapie-infected mice. Molecular Neurobiology. 1994;**8**:105-112

[67] Jeffrey M, McGovern G, Sisó S, González L. Cellular and sub-cellular pathology of animal prion diseases: Relationship between morphological

changes, accumulation of abnormal prion protein and clinical disease. Acta Neuropathologica. 2011;**121**:113-134

[68] DeArmond SJ, Sánchez H, Yehiely F, Qiu Y, Ninchak-Casey A, Daggett V, et al. Selective neuronal targeting in prion disease. Neuron. 1997;**19**:1337-1348

[69] Lawson VA, Collins SJ, Masters CL, Hill AF. Prion protein glycosylation. Journal of Neurochemistry. 2005;**93**:793-801

[70] Beekes M, McBride PA. The spread of prions through the body in naturally acquired transmissible spongiform encephalopathies. The FEBS Journal. 2007;**274**:588-605

[71] Fraser H, Dickinson AG. The sequential development of the brain lesion of scrapie in three strains of mice. Journal of Comparative Pathology. 1968;**78**:301-311

[72] Guentchev M, Wanschitz J, Voigtländer T, Flicker H, Budka H. Selective neuronal vulnerability in human prion diseases. Fatal familial insomnia differs from other types of prion diseases. American Journal of Pathology. 1999;**155**:1453-1457

[73] Somerville RA. How independent are TSE agents from their hosts? Prion. 2013;**7**:272-275. DOI: 10.4161/ pri.25420

[74] Fraser H. Neuropathology of Scrapie: The Precision of Lesion and their Diversity. Slow Transmissible Diseases of the Nervous System. NY: Academic Press; 1979. pp. 387-406

[75] Kim YS, Carp RI, Callahan SM, Natelli M, Wisniewski HM. Vacuolization, incubation period and survival time analyses in three mouse genotypes injected stereotactically in three brain regions

with the 22L scrapie strain. Journal of Neuropathology and Experimental Neurology. 1990;**49**:106-113

[76] Lucassen PJ, Williams A, Chung WCJ, Fraser H. Detection of apoptosis in murine scrapie. Neuroscience Letters. 1995;**198**:185-188

[77] Williams A, Lucassen P, Ritchie D, Bruce M. PrP deposition, microglial activation and neuronal apoptosis in murine scrapie. Experimental Neurology. 1997;**144**:433-438

[78] Fraser J, Halliday W, Brown D, Belichenko P, Jeffrey M. Mechanisms of scrapie-induced neuronal cell death. In: Court L, Dodet B, editors. Transmissible Subacute Spongiform Encephalopathies: Prion Diseases. Paris: Elsevier; 1996. pp. 107-112

[79] Haw JJ, Gray F, Baudrimont M, Escourolle R. Cerebellar changes in 50 cases of Creutzfeldt-Jakob disease with emphasis on granule cell atrophy variant. Acta Neuropathologica. 1981;**7**:196-198

[80] Berciano J, Berciano MT, Polo JM, Figols J, Ciudad J, Lafarga M. Creutzfeldt-Jakob disease with severe involvement of cerebral white matter and cerebellum. Wirschows Archiv. 1990;**417**:533-538

[81] Budka H, Aguzzi A, Brown P, Brucher JM, Bugiani O, Gullotta F, et al. Neuropathological diagnostic criteria for Creutzfeldt-Jakob disease (CJD) and other human spongiform encephalopathies (prion disease). Brain Pathology. 1995;**5**:459-466

[82] Schulz-Schaeffer WJ, Giese A, Windl O, Kretzschmar HA. Polymorphism at codon 129 of the prion protein gene determines cerebellar pathology in Creutzfeldt-Jakob disease. Clinical Neuropathology. 1996;**15**:353-357

[83] Yang Q, Hashizume Y, Yoshida M, Wang Y. Neuropathological study of cerebellar degeneration in prion disease. Neuropathology. 1999;**19**:33-39

[84] Armstrong R, Ironside J, Lantos P, Cairns N. A quantitative study of the pathological changes in the cerebellum in 15 cases of variant Creutzfeldt-Jakob disease (vCJD). Neuropathology and Applied Neurobiology. 2009;**35**:36-45. DOI: 10.1111/j.1365-2990.2008.00979.x

[85] Faucheux B, Morain E, Diouron V, Brandel J, Salomon D, Sazdovitch V, et al. Quantification of surviving cerebellar granule neurons and abnormal prion protein (PrPSc) deposition in sporadic Creutzfeldt-Jakob disease supports a pathogenic role for small PrPSc deposits common to the various molecular subtypes. Neuropathology and Applied Neurobiology. 2011;**37**:500-512. DOI: 10.1111/j.1365-2990.2011.01179.x

[86] Parchi P, Strammiello R, Giese A, Kretzschmar H. Phenotypic variability of sporadic human prion disease and its molecular basis: Past, present and future. Acta Neuropathologica. 2011;**121**:91-112. DOI: 10.1007/s00401-010-0779-6

[87] Cali I, Miller CJ, Parisi J, Geschwind M, Gambetti P, Schonberger L. Distinct pathological phenotypes of Creutzfelds-Jakob disease in recipients of prion-contaminated growth hormone. Acta Neuropathologica. 2015;**3**:37-46

[88] Apps R, Hawkes R. Cerebellar cortical organization: A one-map hypothesis. Nature Reviews. Neuroscience. 2009;**10**:670-681. DOI: 10.1038/nrn2698

[89] Reeber SL, White JJ, Georges-Jones NA, Sillitoe RV. Architecture and development of olivo-cerebellar circuit topography. Frontiers in Neural

Circuits. 2013;**6**:115. DOI: 10.3389/fncir.2012.00115

[90] Brochu G, Maler L, Hawkes R. Zebrin II: A polypeptide antigen expressed selectively by Purkinje cells reveals compartments in rats and fish cerebellum. The Journal of Comparative Neurology. 1990;**291**:538-552

[91] Armstrong R, Cairns N. Spatial patterns of the pathological changes in the cerebellar cortex in sporadic Creutzfeldt-Jakob disease (sCJD). Folia Neuropathologica. 2003;**41**:183-189

[92] Fujita H, Morita N, Furuichi T, Sugihara I. Clustered fine compartmentalization of the mouse embryonic cerebellar cortex and its rearrangement into the postnatal striped configuration. The Journal of Neuroscience. 2012;**32**:15688-15703. DOI: 10.1523/JNEUROSCI.1710-12.2012

[93] Zhou M, Ottenberg G, Sferrazza GF, Lasmézas CI. Highly neurotoxic monomeric alpha-helical prion protein. Proceedings of the National Academy of Sciences of the United States of America. 2012;**109**:3113-3118. DOI: 10.1073/pnas.1118090109

[94] Mallucci G, Ratte S, Asante EA, Linehan J, Gowland I, Jefferys JG, et al. Post-natal knock-out of prion protein alters hippocampal CA1 properties, but does not result in neurodegeneration. The EMBO Journal. 2002;**21**:202-210

[95] Halliday M, Radford H, Mallucci G. Prions: Generation and spread versus neurotoxicity. The Journal of Biological Chemistry. 2014;**289**:19862-19868

[96] Nakagawa T, Zhu H, Morishima N, Li E, Xu J, Bruce A, et al. Caspase-12 mediates endoplasmic reticulum-specific apoptosis and cytotoxicity by amyloid-β. Nature. 2000;**403**:98-103

[97] Hetz C, Russelakis-Carneiro M, Maundrell K, Castilla J, Soto C. Caspase-12 and endoplasmic reticulum stress mediate neurotoxicity of pathological prion protein. The EMBO Journal. 2003;**22**:5435-5445

[98] Soto C, Satani N. The intricate mechanisms of neurodegeneration in priondiseases. Trends in Molecular Medicine. 2011;**17**:14-24

[99] Mukherjee A, Morales-Scheihing D, Gonzalez-Romero D, Green K, Taglialatela G, Soto C. Calcineurin inhibition at the clinical phase of prion disease reduces neurodegeneration, improves behavioral alterations and increases animal survival. PLoS Pathogens. 2010;**6**:e1001138

[100] Sakudo A, Lee DC, Nakamura I, Taniuchi Y, Saeki K, Matsumoto Y, et al. Cell-autonomous PrP-Doppel interaction regulates apoptosis in PrP gene-deficient neuronal cells. Biochemical and Biophysical Research Communications. 2005;**333**:448-454

[101] Kurschner C, Morgan J. The cellular prion protein (PrP) selectively binds to Bcl-2 in the yeast two-hybrid system. Molecular Brain Research. 1995;**30**:165-168

[102] Kurschner C, Morgan J. Analysis of interaction sites in homo- and heteromeric complexes containing Bcl-2 family members and the cellular prion protein. Molecular Brain Research. 1996;**37**:249-258

[103] Laroche-Pierre S, Jodoin J, Leblanc A. Helix 3 is necessary and sufficient for prion protein's anti-Bax function. Journal of Neurochemistry. 2009;**108**:1019-1031

[104] Kuwahara C, Takeuchi AM, Nishimura T, Haraguchi K, Kubosaki A, Matsumoto Y, et al. Prions prevent

neuronal cell-line death. Nature. 1999;**400**:225-226

[105] Kim BH, Lee HG, Choi JK, Kim JI, Choi EK, Carp RI, et al. The cellular prion protein (PrPC) prevents apoptotic neuronal cell death and mitochondrial dysfunction induced by serum deprivation. Brain Research. Molecular Brain Research. 2004;**124**:40-50

[106] Bounhar Y, Zhang Y, Goodyer CG, LeBlanc A. Prion protein protects human neurons against Bax-mediated apoptosis. The Journal of Biological Chemistry. 2001;**276**:39145-39149

[107] Philot T, Drouet B, Pinçon-Raymond M, Vandekerckhove J, Rosseneu M, Chambaz J. A nonfibrillar form of the fusogenic prion protein fragment [118-135] induces apoptotic cell death in rat cortical neurons. Journal of Neurochemistry. 2000;**75**:2298-2308

[108] O'Donovan CN, Tobin D, Cotter TG. Prion protein fragment PrP-(106-126) induces apoptosis via mitochondrial disruption in human neuronal SH-SY5Y cells. The Journal of Biological Chemistry. 2001;**276**:43516-43523

[109] Lin D, Jodoin J, Baril M, Goodyer CG, Leblanc AC. Cytosolic prion protein is the predominant anti-Bax prion protein form: Exclusion of transmembrane and secreted prion protein forms in the anti-Bax function. Biochimica et Biophysica Acta. 2008;**1783**:2001-2012

[110] Giese A, Groschup MH, Hess B, Kretzschmar HA. Neuronal cell death in scrapie-infected mice is due to apoptosis. Brain Pathology. 1995;**5**:213-221

[111] Jesionek-Kupnicka D, Kordek R, Buczyński J, Liberski PP. Apoptosis in relation to neuronal loss in experimental Creutzfeldt-Jakob disease in mice.

Acta Neurobiologiae Experimentalis. 2001;**61**:13-19

[112] Gray F, Chrétien F, Adle-Biassette H, Dorandeu A, Ereau T, Delisle MB, et al. Neuronal apoptosis in Creutzfeldt-Jakob disease. Journal of Neuropathology and Experimental Neurology. 1999;**58**:321-328

[113] Ferrer I. Synaptic pathology and cell death in the cerebellum in Creutzfeldt-Jakob disease. Cerebellum. 2002;**1**:213-222

[114] Drew SC, Haigh CL, Klemm HM, Masters CL, Collins SJ, Barnham KJ, et al. Optical imaging detects apoptosis in the brain and peripheral organs of prion-infected mice. Journal of Neuropathology and Experimental Neurology. 2011;**70**:143-150

[115] Cronier S, Carimalo J, Schaeffer B, Jaumain E, Béringue V, Miquel MC, et al. Endogenous prion protein conversion is required for prion-induced neuritic alterations and neuronal death. The FASEB Journal. 2012;**26**:3854-3861

[116] Sisó S, Puig B, Varea R, Vidal E, Acín C, Prinz M, et al. Abnormal synaptic protein expression and cell death in murine scrapie. Acta Neuropathologica. 2002;**103**:615-626

[117] Falsig J, Sonati T, Herrmann US, Saban D, Li B, Arroyo K, et al. Prion pathogenesis is faithfully reproduced in cerebellar organotypic slice cultures. PLoS Pathogens. 2012;**8**:e1002985

[118] Park SK, Choi SI, Jin JK, Choi EK, Kim JI, Carp RI, et al. Differential expression of Bax and Bcl-2 in the brains of hamsters infected with 263K scrapie agent. Neuroreport. 2000;**11**:1677-1682

[119] Coulpier M, Messiaen S, Hamel R, Fernández de Marco M, Lilin T, Eloit M. Bax deletion does not protect neurons from BSE-induced

death. Neurobiology of Disease. 2006;**23**:603-611

[120] Chiesa R, Piccardo P, Dossena S, Nowoslawski L, Roth KA, Ghetti B, et al. Bax deletion prevents neuronal loss but not neurological symptoms in a transgenic model of inherited prion disease. Proceedings of the National Academy of Sciences of the United States of America. 2005;**102**:238-243

[121] Heitz S, Lutz Y, Rodeau J-L, Zanjani H, Gautheron V, Bombarde G, et al. BAX contributes to Doppel-induced apoptosis of prion protein-deficient Purkinje cells. Developmental Neurobiology. 2007;**67**:670-686

[122] Selimi F, Doughty M, Delhaye-Bouchaud N, Mariani J. Target-related and intrinsic neuronal death in Lurcher mutant mice are both mediated by caspase-3 activation. The Journal of Neuroscience. 2000;**20**:992-1000

[123] Zanjani HS, Vogel MW, Martinou JC, Delhaye-Bouchaud N, Mariani J. Postnatal expression of Hu-bcl-2 gene in Lurcher mutant mice fails to rescue Purkinje cells but protects inferior olivary neurons from target-related cell death. The Journal of Neuroscience. 1998;**18**:319-327

[124] Fan H, Favero M, Vogel MW. Elimination of Bax expression in mice increases cerebellar Purkinje cell numbers but not the number of granule cells. The Journal of Comparative Neurology. 2001;**436**:82-91

[125] Zanjani HS, Vogel MW, Delhaye-Bouchaud N, Martinou JC, Mariani J. Increased cerebellar Purkinje cell numbers in mice overexpressing a human bcl-2 transgene. The Journal of Comparative Neurology. 1996;**374**:332-341

[126] Kim YS, Carp RI, Callahan SM, Wisniewski HM. Incubation periods

and survival times for mice injected stereotaxically with three scrapie strains in different brain regions. The Journal of General Virology. 1987;**68**:695-702

[127] Zanjani HS, Vogel MW, Delhaye-Bouchaud N, Martinou JC, Mariani J. Increased inferior olivary neuron and cerebellar granule cell numbers in transgenic mice overexpressing the human Bcl-2 gene. Journal of Neurobiology. 1997;**32**:502-516

[128] Moore R. Proteomics analysis of amyloid and nonamylois prion disease phenotype reveals both common and divergent mechanisms of neuropathogenesis. Journal of Proteome Research. 2014;**13**:4620-4634

[129] Falsig J, Julius C, Margalith I, Schwarz P, Heppner FL, Aguzzi A. A versatile prion replication assay in organotypic brain slices. Nature Neuroscience. 2008;**11**:109-117

[130] Campeau JL, Wu G, Bell JR, Rasmussen J, Sim VL. Early increase and late decrease of Purkinje cell dendritic spine density in prion-infected organotypic mouse cerebellar cultures. PLoS One. 2013;**8**:e81776

[131] Wolf H, Hossinger A, Fehlinger A, Büttner S, Sim V, McKenzie D, et al. Deposition pattern and subcellular distribution of disease-associated prion protein in cerebellar organotypic slice cultures infected with scrapie. Frontiers in Neuroscience. Nov 4, 2015;**9**:410. DOI: 10.3389/frins.2015.00410

[132] Webb JL, Ravikumar B, Atkins J, Skepper JN, Rubinsztein DC. Alpha-Synuclein is degraded by both autophagy and the proteasome. The Journal of Biological Chemistry. 2003;**278**:25009-25013

[133] Pickford F, Masliah E, Britschgi M, Lucin K, Narasimhan R, Jaeger PA, et al. The autophagy-related protein

beclin 1 shows reduced expression in early Alzheimer disease and regulates amyloid beta accumulation in mice. The Journal of Clinical Investigation. 2008;**118**:2190-2199

[134] Xu Y, Tian C, Wang SB, Xie WL, Guo Y, Zhang J, et al. Activation of the macroautophagic system in scrapie-infected experimental animals and human genetic prion diseases. Autophagy. 2012;**8**:1604-1620

[135] Heitz S, Grant NJ, Leschiera R, Haeberlé AM, Demais V, Bombarde G, et al. Autophagy and cell death of Purkinje cells overexpressing Doppel in Ngsk Prnp-deficient mice. Brain Pathology. 2010;**20**:119-132

[136] Petersén A, Larsen KE, Behr GG, Romero N, Przedborski S, Brundin P, et al. Expanded CAG repeats in exon 1 of the Huntington's disease gene stimulate dopamine-mediated striatal neuron autophagy and degeneration. Human Molecular Genetics. 2001;**10**:1243-1254

[137] Nixon RA. Autophagy, amyloidogenesis and Alzheimer disease. Journal of Cell Science. 2007;**120**:4081-4091

[138] Spilman P, Podlutskaya N, Hart MJ, Debnath J, Gorostiza O, Bredesen D, et al. Inhibition of mTOR by rapamycin abolishes cognitive deficits and reduces amyloid-beta levels in a mouse model of Alzheimer's disease. PLoS One. 2010;**5**:e9979

[139] Yang DS, Stavrides P, Mohan PS, Kaushik S, Kumar A, Ohno M, et al. Therapeutic effects of remediating autophagy failure in a mouse model of Alzheimer disease by enhancing lysosomal proteolysis. Autophagy. 2011;**7**:788-789

[140] Heiseke A, Aguib Y, Riemer C, Baier M, Schätzl HM. Lithium induces clearance of protease resistant prion protein in prion-infected cells by induction of autophagy. Journal of Neurochemistry. 2009;**109**:25-34

[141] Cortes CJ, Qin K, Cook J, Solanki A, Mastrianni JA. Rapamycin delays disease onset and prevents PrP plaque deposition in a mouse model of Gerstmann-Sträussler-Scheinker disease. The Journal of Neuroscience. 2012;**32**:12396-12405

[142] Cuervo AM, Stefanis L, Fredenburg R, Lansbury PT, Sulzer D. Impaired degradation of mutant alpha-synuclein by chaperone-mediated autophagy. Science. 2004;**305**:1292-1295

[143] Chu C. Autophagic stress in neuronal injury and disease. Journal of Neuropathology and Experimental Neurology. 2006;**65**:423-432

[144] Kovacs G, Budka H. Prion diseases: From protein to cell pathology. The American Journal of Pathology. 2008;**172**:555-565

[145] Boelaard JW, Schlote W, Tateishi J. Neuronal autophagy in experimental Creutzfeldt-Jakob's disease. Acta Neuropathologica. 1989;**78**:410-418

[146] Dron M, Bailly Y, Beringue V, Haeberlé AM, Griffond B, Risold PY, et al. Scrg1 is induced in TSE and brain injuries, and associated with autophagy. The European Journal of Neuroscience. 2005;**22**:133-146

[147] Dron M, Bailly Y, Beringue V, Haeberlé A-M, Griffond B, Risold P-Y, et al. SCRG1, a potential marker of autophagy in transmissible spongiform encephalopathies. Autophagy. 2006;**2**:58-60

[148] Oh JM, Shin HY, Park SJ, Kim BH, Choi JK, Choi EK, et al. The involvement of cellular prion protein in the autophagy pathway in neuronal cells. Molecular and Cellular Neurosciences. 2008;**39**:238-247

[149] Doh-Ura K, Iwaki T, Caughey B. Lysosomotropic agents and cysteine protease inhibitors inhibit scrapie-associated prion protein accumulation. Journal of Virology. 2000;**74**:4894-4897

[150] Beranger F, Crozet C, Goldsborough A, Lehmann S. Trehalose impairs aggregation of PrPSc molecules and protects prion-infected cells against oxidative damage. Biochemical and Biophysical Research Communications. 2008;**374**:44-48. DOI: 10.1016/j.bbrc.2008.06.094

[151] Heiseke A, Aguib Y, Schätzl H. Autophagy, prion infection and their mutual interactions. Current Issues in Molecular Biology. 2010;**12**:11

[152] Yun SW, Ertmer A, Flechsig E, Gilch S, Riederer P, Gerlach M, et al. The tyrosine kinase inhibitor imatinib mesylate delays prion neuroinvasion by inhibiting prion propagation in the periphery. Journal of Neurovirology. 2007;**13**:328-337

[153] Aguib Y, Heiseke A, Gilch S, Riemer C, Baier M, Schätzl HM, et al. Autophagy induction by trehalose counteracts cellular prion infection. Autophagy. 2009;**5**:361-369

[154] Zhou M, Ottenberg G, Sferrazza GF, Hubbs C, Fallahi M, Rumbaugh G, et al. Neuronal death induced by misfolded prion protein is due to NAD+ depletion and can be relieved in vitro and in vivo by NAD+ replenishment. Brain. 2015;**138**:992-1008. DOI: 10.1093/brain/awv002

[155] Weissmann C, Flechsig E. PrP knock-out and PrP transgenic mice in prion research. British Medical Bulletin. 2003;**66**:43-60

[156] Criado JR, Sánchez-Alavez M, Conti B, Giacchino JL, Wills DN, Henriksen SJ, et al. Mice devoid of prion protein have cognitive deficits that

are rescued by reconstitution of PrP in neurons. Neurobiology of Disease. 2005;**19**:255-265

[157] Oh JM, Choi EK, Carp RI, Kim YS. Oxidative stress impairs autophagic flux in prion protein-deficient hippocampal cells. Autophagy. 2018:1448-1461

[158] Shin HY, Park JH, Carp RI, Choi EK, Kim YS. Deficiency of prion protein induces impaired autophagic flux in neurons. Frontiers in Aging Neuroscience. 2014;**6**:207. DOI: 10.3389/fnagi.2014.00207

[159] Ko DC, Milenkovic L, Beier SM, Manuel H, Buchanan J, Scott MP. Cell-autonomous death of cerebellar purkinje neurons with autophagy in Niemann-pick type C disease. PLoS Genetics. 2005;**1**:81-95

[160] Sanchez-Varo R, Trujillo-Estrada L, Sanchez-Mejias E, Torres M, Baglietto-Vargas D, Moreno-Gonzalez I, et al. Abnormal accumulation of autophagic vesicles correlates with axonal and synaptic pathology in young Alzheimer's mice hippocampus. Acta Neuropathologica. 2012;**123**:53-70. DOI: 10.1007/s00401-011-0896-x

[161] Sakaguchi S, Katamine S, Nishida N, Moriuchi R, Shigematsu K, Sugimoto T, et al. Loss of cerebellar Purkinje cells in aged mice homozygous for a disrupted PrP gene. Nature. 1996;**380**:528-531

[162] Katamine S, Nishida N, Sugimoto T, Noda T, Sakaguchi S, Shigematsu K, et al. Impaired motor coordination in mice lacking prion protein. Cellular and Molecular Neurobiology. 1998;**18**:731-732

[163] Rossi D, Cozzio A, Flechsig E, Klein MA, Rulicke T, Aguzzi A, et al. Onset of ataxia and Purkinje cell loss in PrP null mice inversely correlated with

Dpl level in brain. The EMBO Journal. 2001;**20**:694-702

[164] Weissmann C, Aguzzi A. PrP's double causes trouble. Science. 1999;**286**:914-915

[165] Moore RC, Lee IY, Silverman GL, Harrison PM, Strome R, Heinrich C, et al. Ataxia in prion protein (PrP)-deficient mice is associated with upregulation of the novel PrP-like protein doppel. Journal of Molecular Biology. 1999;**292**:797-817

[166] Lu K, Wang W, Xie Z, Wong B-S, Li R, Petersen RB, et al. Structural characterization of the recombinant human doppel protein. Biochemistry. 2000;**39**:13575-13583

[167] Moore RC, Mastrangelo P, Bouzamondo E, Heinrich C, Legname G, Prusiner SB, et al. Doppel-induced cerebellar degeneration in transgenic mice. Proceedings of the National Academy of Sciences of the United States of America. 2001;**98**:15288-15293

[168] Lemaire-Vieille C, Bailly Y, Erlich P, Loeuillet C, Brocard J, Haeberlé AM, et al. Ataxia with cerebellar lesions in mice expressing chimeric PrP-Dpl protein. The Journal of Neuroscience. 2013;**33**:1391-1399

[169] Watts JC, Westaway D. The prion protein family: Diversity, rivalry, and dysfunction. Biochimica et Biophysica Acta. 2007;**1772**:654-672

[170] Heitz S, Gautheron V, Lutz Y, Rodeau JL, Zanjani HS, Sugihara I, et al. Bcl-2 conteracts Doppel-induced apoptosis of prion protein-deficient Purkinje cells in the Ngsk *Prnp*$^{0/0}$ mouse. Developmental Neurobiology. 2008;**68**:332-348

[171] Heitz S, Grant NJ, Bailly Y. Doppel induces autophagic stress in prion protein-deficient Purkinje cells. Autophagy. 2009;**5**:422-424

[172] Ding W, Yin X. Sorting, recognition and activation of the misfolded protein degradation pathways through macroautophagy and the proteasome. Autophagy. 2008;**16**:141-150

[173] Wang QJ, Ding Y, Kohtz DS, Mizushima N, Cristea IM, Rout MP, et al. Induction of autophagy in axonal dystrophy and degeneration. The Journal of Neuroscience. 2006;**26**:8057-8068

[174] Yue Z. Regulation of neuronal autophagy in axon: Implication of autophagy in axonal function and dysfunction/degeneration. Autophagy. 2007;**3**:139-141

[175] Yue Z, Friedman L, Komatsu M, Tanaka K. The cellular pathways of neuronal autophagy and their implication in neurodegenerative diseases. Biochimica et Biophysica Acta. 2009;**1793**:1496-1507

[176] Maday S, Wallace KE, Holzbaur EL. Autophagosomes initiate distally and mature during transport toward the cell soma in primary neurons. The Journal of Cell Biology. 2012;**196**:407-417

[177] Nixon RA, Yang DS, Lee JH. Neurodegenerative lysosomal disorders: A continuum from development to late age. Autophagy. 2008;**4**:590-599

[178] Fimia G, Piacentini M. Regulation of autophagy in mammals and its interplay with apoptosis. Cellular and Molecular Life Sciences. 2010;**67**:1581-1588. DOI: 10.1007/s00018-010-0284-z

[179] Metzger F, Kapfhammer JP. Protein kinase C: Its role in activity-dependent Purkinje cell dendritic development and plasticity. Cerebellum. 2003;**2**:206-214

[180] Dole S, Heitz S, Bombarde G, Haeberlé A-M, Demais V, Grant NJ, et al.

New insights into Doppel neurotoxicity
using cerebellar organotypic cultures
from prion protein-deficient mice. In:
Medimond International Proceedings,
Monduzzi Editors. Bologna Prion 2010,
Salzburg, Austria. Sep 08-11, 2010.
pp. 7-14

Chapter 3

A Molecular Mechanism for Abnormal Prion Protein Accumulation

Keiji Uchiyama and Suehiro Sakaguchi

Abstract

A fundamental event in the pathogenesis of prion disease is the conversion of cellular prion protein into an abnormally folded isoform (PrP^{Sc}), which is the infectious causative agent of disease. With progression of disease, PrP^{Sc} is replicated and excessively accumulated in most cases. However, the molecular mechanism for excessive accumulation of PrP^{Sc} is not well understood. Recently, Sortilin, a member of the VPS10P domain receptor family, has been identified as a sorting receptor that directs prion protein (PrP) to the lysosomal degradation pathway. Moreover, it has been shown that prion infection impairs Sortilin function, resulting in delayed PrP^{Sc} degradation. In this chapter, we explain the mechanisms for PrP trafficking into the lysosomal degradation pathway mediated by Sortilin and overaccumulation of PrP^{Sc} caused by Sortilin dysfunction.

Keywords: PrP^{Sc}, PrP^{Sc} accumulation, PrP^{Sc} degradation, Sortilin, sorting, VPS10P domain, sorting receptor, VPS10P domain receptor

1. Introduction

Prion diseases are a group of fatal neurodegenerative disorders that are caused by the transmissible misfolded isoform (PrP^{Sc}) of the cellular prion (PrP^{C}) [1], including Creutzfeldt-Jakob disease of humans, bovine spongiform encephalopathy, and scrapie of sheep. PrP^{Sc} is a β-sheet rich conformer of PrP^{C} and is partially resistant to protease. With progression of prion disease, PrP^{Sc} is replicated and accumulated in the brain, and neuronal dysfunction and death occur. Previous studies have shown that PrP-null mice neither develop the disease nor accumulate PrP^{Sc} even after prions are inoculated into their brains [2, 3]. This indicates that replication and accumulation of PrP^{Sc} are closely related to the pathogenesis of prion disease. Therefore, elucidation of the mechanisms of PrP^{Sc} degradation and accumulation is critical for understanding the pathogenic mechanism of prion disease and for developing therapeutic agents.

PrP^{Sc} usually accumulates excessively over PrP^{C} in cultured cells and mouse brains (**Figure 1**). This strongly indicates that PrP^{Sc} is protected against its proteolytic degradation. Actually, several studies have reported that the proteolytic systems (e.g., lysosomal degradation and ubiquitin-proteasomal degradation systems) are inhibited by prion infection [4–7], and PrP^{Sc} is found at the cell surface and in endosomal/lysosomal compartments [8–10]. Moreover, when PrP^{Sc} was

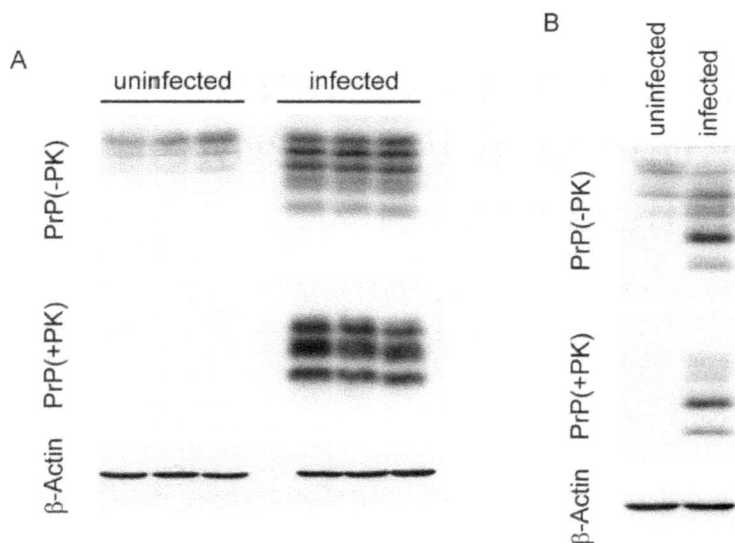

Figure 1.
PrP expression in mice brain and N2a cells. (A) Total PrP and PrP^Sc were compared between RML prion infected mouse brains at terminal stage and age matched uninfected mice brain by western blotting. (B) N2a cells were treated with uninfected or 22 L-prion infected mice brain homogenate. At 30 dpi, total PrP and PrP^Sc were detected by western blotting. Blots were probed with anti-PrP antibody (6D11) and anti-β-actin antibody.

fractionated by detergent-based biochemical fractionation, most of the PrP^{Sc} was detected in detergent-resistant membrane (DRM) fractions [11], suggesting that PrP^{Sc} mainly exists in membrane bound form and PrP^{Sc} is degraded preferentially in lysosomes, but not by cytosolic proteasomes. PrP^{Sc} to be degraded in lysosomes might be preferentially selected and directed into the lysosomal degradation pathway by dedicated membrane trafficking machinery. Therefore, knowledge of the mechanism that sorts PrP into late endosomal/lysosomal compartments should be important for understanding the accumulation of PrP^{Sc}.

2. PrP^{Sc} accumulation

Figure 1A shows the expression of total PrP and PrP^{Sc} in uninfected and prion-infected mouse brains. In this figure, we can easily recognize that the total amount of PrP in infected mouse brains is larger than in uninfected mouse brains. In cultured cells, such excessive expression of total PrP in infected cells was also confirmed (**Figure 1B**). These results indicate that the amount of PrP^{Sc} in infected cells is larger than PrP^C in uninfected cells, and that PrP^{Sc} is protected against proteolytic degradation.

Why is PrP^{Sc} protected from proteolysis and over-accumulated? One possible reason is the protease resistance of PrP^{Sc} that is attributed to its β-rich structure at the C-terminal region. If such protease resistance mainly affected the inhibition of PrP^{Sc} degradation, most of the PrP^{Sc} could be found in the lysosome, which contains various kinds of hydrolytic enzymes and is a major compartment responsible for the digestion of macromolecules such as proteins. The majority of PrP^{Sc} is actually observed intracellularly, whereas PrP^C mainly localizes to the cell surface (**Figure 2A**). However, detailed analyses of its intracellular distribution show that PrP^{Sc} is widely distributed in posttrans Golgi network (TGN) compartments [8–10] (**Figure 2B**). From these

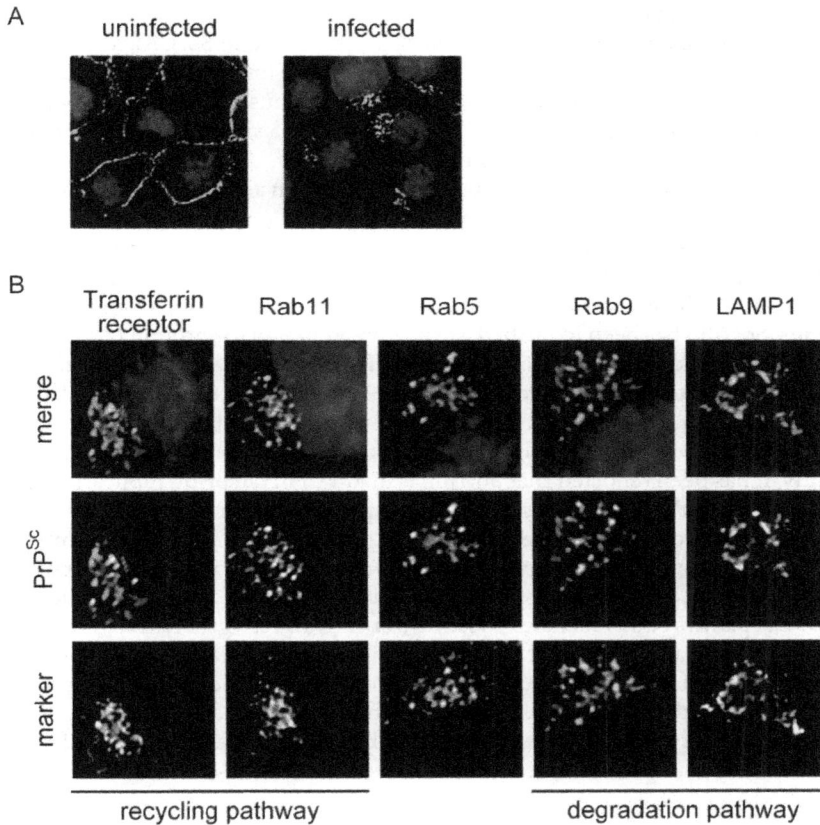

Figure 2.
PrP^{Sc} is widely distributed in post-Golgi compartments. (A) PrP^{C} (green, uninfected cells) and PrP^{Sc} (green, infected cells) were visualized by immunofluorescence staining with mouse monoclonal anti-PrP antibody (SAF83) and anti-PrP^{Sc} antibody (132), respectively. (B) PrP^{Sc} indicated organelle markers in prion infected cells were doubly stained with anti-PrP^{Sc} antibody (132) and anti-transferrin receptor, Rab11, Rab5, Rab9 and LAMP1 antibody, respectively. DAPI was used for nuclear stain (blue).

observations, it seems that impairment of PrP^{Sc} trafficking into lysosomes as well as its protease-resistance causes inhibition of degradation and over-accumulation of PrP^{Sc}.

3. Sortilin and other VPS10P domain receptors

PrP would have to move by transport vesicles in post-TGN compartments, including TGN, endosomes, lysosomes, and the plasma membrane. Then, in this transport network, the PrP to be degraded could be sorted into transport carriers bound for late endosomal/lysosomal compartments. For this purpose, a sorting receptor might be useful and required because it can select and concentrate a target cargo protein into transport carriers and promote transport carrier formation. In our recent study, Sortilin has been identified as a sorting receptor that directs PrP into late endosomal/lysosomal compartments. Sortilin is a member of the VPS10P domain receptor family, which is comprised of five members (Sortilin, SorCS1, SorCS2, SorCS3, and SorLA). In this section, briefly, we describe Sortilin and other VPS10P receptors and their implications for neurodegenerative diseases.

VPS10P-domain receptors are multiligand type-I transmembrane proteins. They contain five members, Sortilin, SorLA, SorCS1, SorCS2, and SorCS3, and deliver a number of target cargo proteins to their destinations, interacting with them via VPS10P domains on the luminal/extracellular N-terminus (**Figure 3**). The whole luminal/extracellular region in Sortilin is composed of a simple VPS10P domain, but other receptors have additional modules (**Figure 3**).

VPS10P-domain receptors are expressed in the brain and are involved in neuronal function and viability [12, 13]. Sortilin binds to progranulin and mediates endocytosis and delivery of progranulin into lysosomes [14], and rare nonsynonymous variants in SORT1 increase the risk for frontotemporal lobar degeneration [15]. Sortilin also mediates trafficking of neuronal degeneration causative and related proteins. Sortilin has been identified as an amyloid precursor protein (APP) interaction partner and promotes α-cleavage of APP [16]. In addition, Sortilin interacts with BACE1, β-site APP cleavage enzyme 1, and mediates its retrograde trafficking from the plasma membrane to TGN via early endosomes [17]. It has been suggested that Sortilin is potentially associated with Parkinson's disease [18]. Moreover, recently, it has been reported that Sortilin is involved in tau prion replication [19].

As for other VPS10P receptors, it has been reported that SorLA is associated with sporadic and late-onset Alzheimer's disease (AD) [5, 20]. SorLA directs APP into the recycling pathway and protects APP from β-cleavage resulting in Aβ generation [5, 21, 22]. On the other hand, loss of SorLA shifts the traffic flow of APP to the late endosomal pathway and facilitates β-cleavage of APP and Aβ-generation [5, 21, 22]. In addition, a meta-analysis indicated that multiple SorLA variants are associated with the risk of Alzheimer's disease [23]. SorCS1 is also involved in APP transport and Aβ-generation and is identified as a risk factor for Alzheimer's disease [24, 25]. Variants of SorCS2 and SorCS3 are also associated with the risk of Alzheimer's disease [24, 25]. Although a number of studies have indicated that VPS10P-domain receptors are

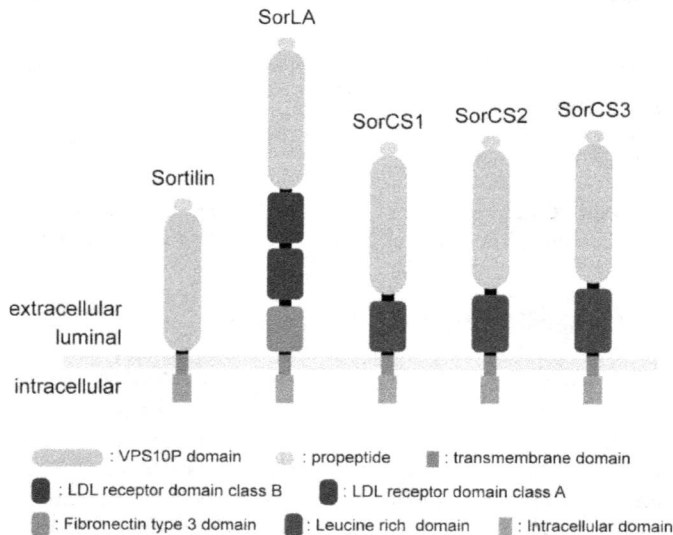

Figure 3.
VPS10P domain receptors. VPS10P-domain receptors are multiligand type-I transmembrane proteins. They contain five members, Sortilin, SorLA, SorCS1, SorCS2 and SorCS3. The extracellular/luminal region of VPS10P receptors contains VPS10P domain and additional domains. The intracellular domain of VPS10P receptors contains motifs for interaction with adaptor proteins. The propeptide at N-terminal region is cleaved by furin in the TGN.

implicated in neurodegenerative diseases and their impairment could be a risk factor for diseases, the relation between VPS10P receptors and prion disease is not known.

4. Role of Sortilin in PrP trafficking

Sortilin has been identified as a novel PrP-binding protein and is colocalized with PrP^C both at the cell surface and intracellular compartments [11]. In Sortilin-knockdown (Sortilin-KD) uninfected cells, most of the PrP^C is localized at the cell surface, and PrP^C expression is increased. In addition, a PrP^C uptake experiment, in which cell surface PrP^C was labeled with anti-PrP antibody and internalized labeled PrP^C was measured after incubation, demonstrated that PrP^C internalization was weakened by Sortilin-KD [11]. These results indicate that Sortilin acts as a cell surface receptor for PrP^C endocytosis.

PrP^C was also colocalized with Sortilin intracellularly [11]. This made us recollect that Sortilin could function intracellularly as a sorting receptor for PrP trafficking. When the internalized labeled PrP^C was costained for either Rab9 (a late endosomal marker) or Rab11 (a recycling endosomal marker) by indirect immunofluorescence, the internalized PrP^C distributed to both late and recycling endosomes in control cells, whereas, in Sortilin-depleted cells, it failed to localize to late endosomes, and most of the internalized PrP^C is localized to recycling endosomes [11]. These observations indicate that Sortilin is also required for sorting of PrP^C into late endosomes to degrade it.

Moreover, when wild type (wt) and Sortilin-knockout (ΔSort) cells were treated with NH$_4$Cl, which increases lysosomal pH and inhibits proteolytic enzymes in lysosomes, PrP^C was effectively accumulated in wt but not in ΔSort cells [11], and PrP^C colocalization with LAMP1, a lysosomal marker, in NH$_4$Cl-treated ΔSort cells was significantly lower than NH$_4$Cl-treated wt cells [11]. These results suggest that ΔSort cells failed to transport PrP^C properly into lysosomes.

Altogether, it could be concluded that Sortilin functions as a cell surface receptor for PrP^C internalization and a sorting receptor to direct PrP^C to lysosomes via late endosomes (**Figure 4**). We would be able to extend such a role of Sortilin in PrP^C trafficking to PrP^{Sc} because Sortilin directly interacted with PrP^C through its highly flexible N-terminal domain and anti-Sortilin antibody coprecipitated both PrP^C and PrP^{Sc}. In practical terms, Sortilin is implicated in PrP^{Sc} degradation.

The inhibition of Sortilin inhibited PrP^C internalization by ~20% in the PrP^C uptake assay [11]. This result raises a question. Why is PrP^C endocytosis inhibited partially even when Sortilin function is almost or completely abolished [11]? There are suggestive findings to answer this question. We examined the PrP distribution in uninfected wt cells and in uninfected ΔSort cells by detergent-based biochemical fractionation. Sixty three percent of PrP^C in wt cells was detected in detergent resistant membrane (DRM) fractions, generally recognized as raft fractions, but thirty-seven percent of PrP^C was also found in detergent soluble (nonraft) fractions [11]. Sortilin deficiency changed the PrP^C distribution, and PrP^C in nonraft fractions was reduced to ~15% in ΔSort cells [11]. At present, it is thought that both lipid raft- and clathrin-mediated endocytosis execute PrP^C internalization [13, 26]. Sortilin was mostly isolated in nonraft fractions [11]. It has been reported that the cytoplasmic tail of Sortilin can interact with clathrin-associated adaptor protein complex, AP-2, at the plasma membrane and facilitate clathrin-mediated endocytosis [13, 27, 28]. We showed that the recombinant PrP devoid of its N-terminal domain (residues 23–88) (PrPΔ23–88) did not bind to Sortilin. Additionally, internalization and lysosomal degradation of PrPΔ23–88 were inhibited, and it accumulated at the cell surface [11]. These results are in good agreement with a previous report: the

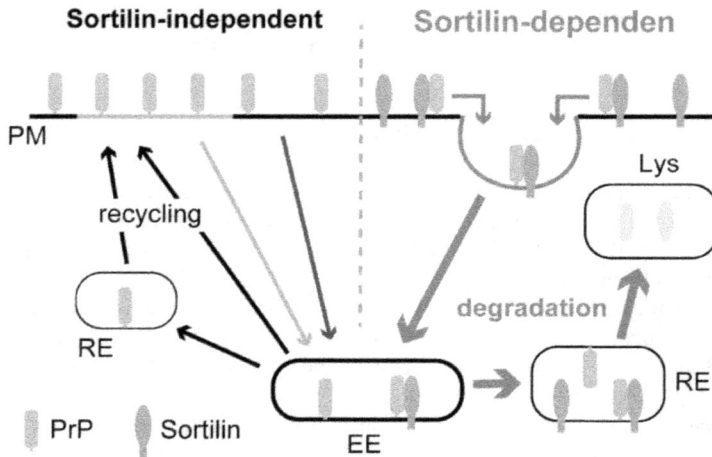

Figure 4.
Role of Sortilin in PrP-trafficking. Sortilin internalizes PrP from nonraft domain and direct into late endosomal/lysosomal degradation pathway. PrP internalized from lipid raft domain in Sortilin-independent manner would be largely recycled into cell surface. PrP might be also internalized from nonraft domain in Sortilin-independent manner. Red arrows indicate Sortilin mediated PrP-trafficking pathway. Blue line is lipid raft domain. EE: Early endosome, LE: Late endosomes, RE: Recycling endosomes, Lys: Lysosomes, PM: Plasma membrane.

N-terminal domain (residues 23–107) of PrP^C is sufficient for its endocytosis mediated by clathrin [29]. It is therefore inferred that Sortilin internalizes PrP^C from nonraft domains at the cell surface by clathrin-coated vesicles. Moreover, it has been shown that the expression of total PrP^C was not changed even when the flotillin-1–mediated lipid raft-dependent endocytosis of PrP^C was inhibited by the knockdown of flotillin-1 [30]. Their and our results suggest that Sortilin-mediated endocytosis directs PrP^C into the late endosomal/lysosomal degradation pathway, whereas PrP^C that is internalized from the lipid raft domain in a Sortilin-independent manner largely enters the recycling pathway (**Figure 4**).

5. Dysfunction of Sortilin by prion infection

Sortilin expression also affects PrP^{Sc} levels. Sortilin-KD increased PrP^{Sc} in prion infected cells, similarly to PrP^C in uninfected cells [11]. On the contrary, overexpression of Sortilin in infected cells reduced PrP^{Sc} [11]. Furthermore, when we investigated PrP^{Sc} accumulation in $Sort1^{+/+}$ and $Sort1^{-/-}$ mouse brains after intracerebral prion inoculation, PrP^{Sc} levels in $Sort1^{-/-}$ mouse brains were significantly higher than in $Sort1^{+/+}$ mouse brains at the early stages of disease (at 45, 60, 90 dpi) [11], suggesting an inhibition of PrP^{Sc} degradation. Namely, dysfunction of Sortilin causes excessive accumulation. If so, does prion infection inhibit Sortilin function? Notably, Sortilin in infected cells was ~50% lower than in uninfected cells [11]. Moreover, in infected mouse brains at terminal stage, Sortilin also fell to ~45% as compared with age-matched uninfected mice [11]. These observations suggested that prion infection downregulated Sortilin expression. To confirm this, uninfected cells were treated with RML prion-infected mouse brain homogenate, and Sortilin and PrP^{Sc} in individual cells were visualized by double immunofluorescence staining at 9 dpi (**Figure 5**). In cells displaying bright green signals derived from PrP^{Sc}, little Sortilin (red) was detected, whereas the bright red fluorescence of Sortilin was observed in the others; that is, Sortilin expression was reduced by prion infection.

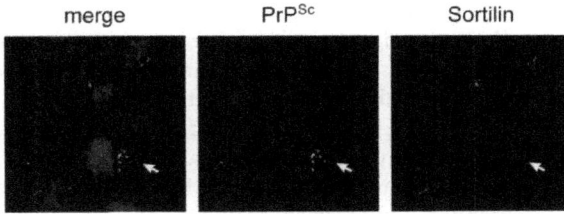

Figure 5.
Prion infection reduces Sortilin expression. Immunofluorescence staining of Sortilin (red) and PrP^{Sc} (green) 9 days after infection of uninfected cells with RML prions. Four horizontal serial images at 1 μm interval were collected, and orthogonally projected image was created. DAPI was used for nuclear stain (blue). Yellow arrow indicates PrP^{Sc}-positive cell.

To clarify why Sortilin is reduced by prion infection, we examined mRNA transcript levels by RT-PCR. There was little difference in Sortilin mRNA abundance between uninfected and infected cells. This suggested that the degradation of Sortilin was facilitated in prion infected cells. Hence, we treated cells with inhibitors of proteolytic degradation. The expression of Sortilin was almost the same in both untreated and MG132-treated cells but increased in NH$_4$Cl-treated cells [11]. In particular, Sortilin expression was dramatically improved in NH$_4$Cl-treated prion-infected cells, and another lysosomal inhibitor, concanamycin A, also improved Sortilin expression in infected cells [11], suggesting that Sortilin is over-degraded in prion-infected cells in lysosomes.

6. Conclusions

Sortilin has been identified as a novel PrP-binding protein and functions as a sorting receptor to direct PrP into late endosomal/lysosomal compartments.

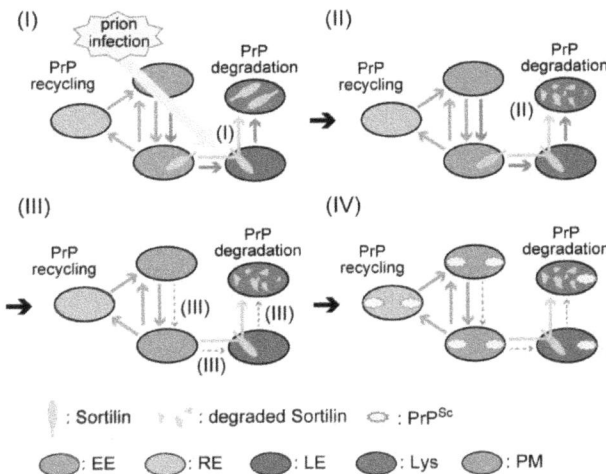

Figure 6.
Possible mechanism for PrP^{Sc} over-accumulation by prion infection. (I) the entry of Sortilin into the lysosomal degradation pathway is facilitated (green arrow) by prion infection (yellow arrow), (II) Sortilin is over-degraded in lysosomes, (III) trafficking of PrP^{Sc} to late endosomal/lysosomal compartments is restricted (red broken arrow), and (IV) PrP^{Sc} is protected against its degradation in lysosomes and is excessively accumulated. Red arrows indicate Sortilin-mediated PrP-trafficking pathway and blue arrows indicate other PrP-trafficking pathways. EE: Early endosomes, LE: Late endosomes, RE: Recycling endosomes, Lys: Lysosomes, PM: Plasma membrane.

Dysfunction of Sortilin induces delayed degradation and excessive accumulation of PrP. Notably, prion infection downregulated Sortilin expression by facilitating Sortilin degradation in lysosomes. Finally, we summarize a possible mechanism of excessive accumulation of PrP^{Sc} during prion infection (**Figure 6**): (I) the entry of Sortilin into the lysosomal degradation pathway is facilitated by prion infection, (II) Sortilin is over-degraded in lysosomes, (III) trafficking of PrP^{Sc} to late endosomal/lysosomal compartments is restricted, and (IV) PrP^{Sc} is protected against its degradation in lysosomes and is excessively accumulated. However, it still remains unclear how prion infection facilitates Sortilin degradation in lysosomes.

Acknowledgements

This work was supported by the following: Pilot Research Support Program in Tokushima University received by KU; Naito Foundation received by KU; JSPS KAKENHI grant (grant No. 26460557, received by KU; MEXT KAKENHI grant (grant No, 17H05702, received by KU; JSPS KAKENHI grant (grant No. 26293212, received by SS; MEXT KAKENHI grant (grant No, 15H01560 and 17H05701, received by SS; and Practical Research Project for Rare/Intractable Diseases of the Japan Agency for Medical Research and Development (AMED) received by SS.

Conflict of interest

The authors have declared that no competing interests exist.

Author details

Keiji Uchiyama* and Suehiro Sakaguchi*
Institute for Advanced Medical Sciences, Tokushima University, Tokushima, Japan

*Address all correspondence to: ku200@tokishima-u.ac.jp and sakaguchi@tokushima-u.ac.jp

IntechOpen

References

[1] Prusiner SB. Prions. Proceedings of the National Academy of Sciences of the United States of America. 1998;**95**(23):13363-13383

[2] Büeler H, Aguzzi A, Sailer A, Greiner RA, Autenried P, Aguet M, Weissmann C. Mice devoid of PrP are resistant to scrapie. Cell. 1993;**73**(7):1339-1347

[3] Sakaguchi S, Katamine S, Shigematsu K, Nakatani A, Moriuchi R, Nishida N, Kurokawa K, Nakaoke R, Sato H, Jishage K. Accumulation of proteinase K-resistant prion protein (PrP) is restricted by the expression level of normal PrP in mice inoculated with a mouse-adapted strain of the Creutzfeldt-Jakob disease agent. Journal of Virology. 1995;**69**(12):7586-7592

[4] Kristiansen M, Deriziotis P, Dimcheff DE, Jackson GS, Ovaa H, Naumann H, Clarke AR, van Leeuwen FWB, Menendez-Benito V, Dantuma NP, Portis JL, Collinge J, Tabrizi SJ. Disease-associated prion protein oligomers inhibit the 26S proteasome. Molecular Cell. 2007;**26**(2):175-188

[5] Rogaeva E, Meng Y, Lee JH, Gu Y, Kawarai T, Zou F, Katayama T, Baldwin CT, Cheng R, Hasegawa H, Chen F, Shibata N, Lunetta KL, Pardossi-Piquard R, Bohm C, Wakutani Y, Adrienne Cupples L, Cuenco KT, Green RC, Pinessi L, Rainero I, Sorbi S, Bruni A, Duara R, Graff-Radford N, Petersen R, Dickson D, Der SD, Fraser PE, Schmitt-Ulms G, Younkin S, Mayeux R, Farrer LA, St George-Hyslop P. The neuronal sortilin-related receptor SORL1 is genetically associated with Alzheimer's disease. Nature Genetics. 2007;**39**(2):168-177

[6] Andre R, Tabrizi SJ. Misfolded PrP and a novel mechanism of proteasome inhibition. Prion. 2012;**6**(1):32-36

[7] Shim SY, Karri S, Law S, Schatzl HM, Gilch S. Prion infection impairs lysosomal degradation capacity by interfering with rab7 membrane attachment in neuronal cells. Scientific Reports. 2016;**6**:21658

[8] Uchiyama K, Muramatsu N, Yano M, Usui T, Miyata H, Sakaguchi S. Prions disturb post-Golgi trafficking of membrane proteins. Nature Communications. 2013;**4**:1846

[9] Yamasaki T, Suzuki A, Shimizu T, Watarai M, Hasebe R, Horiuchi M. Characterization of intracellular localization of PrP Sc in prion-infected cells using a mAb that recognizes the region consisting of aa 119-127 of mouse PrP. The Journal of General Virology. 2012;**93**(3):668-680

[10] Veith NM, Plattner H, Stuermer CAO, Schulz-Schaeffer WJ, Bürkle A. Immunolocalisation of PrPSc in scrapie-infected N2a mouse neuroblastoma cells by light and electron microscopy. European Journal of Cell Biology. 2009;**88**(1):45-63

[11] Uchiyama K, Tomita M, Yano M, Chida J, Hara H, Das NR, Nykjaer A, Sakaguchi S. Prions amplify through degradation of the VPS10P sorting receptor sortilin. PLoS Pathogens. 2017;**13**(6):e1006470

[12] Nykjaer A, Lee R, Teng KK, Jansen P. Sortilin is essential for proNGF-induced neuronal cell death. Nature. 2004;**427**:15-20

[13] Nykjaer A, Willnow TE. Sortilin: A receptor to regulate neuronal viability and function. Trends in Neurosciences. 2012;**35**(4):261-270

[14] Hu F, Padukkavidana T, Vagter CB, Brady OA, Zheng Y, Mackenzie IR, Feldman HH, Nykjaer A, Strittmatter SM. Sortilin-mediated endocytosis

determines levels of the frontotemporal dementia protein, progranulin. Neuron. 2010;**68**(4):654-667

[15] Philtjens S, Van Mossevelde S, van der Zee J, Wauters E, Dillen L, Vandenbulcke M, Vandenberghe R, Ivanoiu A, Sieben A, Willems C, Benussi L, Ghidoni R, Binetti G, Borroni B, Padovani A, Pastor P, Diez-Fairen M, Aguilar M, de Mendonça A, Miltenberger-Miltényi G, Hernández I, Boada M, Ruiz A, Nacmias B, Sorbi S, Almeida MR, Santana I, Clarimón J, Lleó A, Frisoni GB, Sanchez-Valle R, Lladó A, Gómez-Tortosa E, Gelpi E, Van den Broeck M, Peeters K, Cras P, De Deyn PP, Engelborghs S, Cruts M, Van Broeckhoven C, BELNEU Consortium, and EU EOD Consortium. Rare nonsynonymous variants in SORT1 are associated with increased risk for frontotemporal dementia. Neurobiology of Aging. 2018;**66**:181.e3-181.e10

[16] Gustafsen C, Glerup S, Pallesen LT, Olsen D, Andersen OM, Nykjaer A, Madsen P, Petersen CM. Sortilin and SorLA display distinct roles in processing and trafficking of amyloid precursor protein. The Journal of Neuroscience. 2013;**33**(1):64-71

[17] Finan GM, Okada H, Kim T-W. BACE1 retrograde trafficking is uniquely regulated by the cytoplasmic domain of sortilin. The Journal of Biological Chemistry. 2011;**286**(14):12602-12616

[18] Dhungel N, Eleuteri S, Li L, Kramer NJ, Chartron JW, Spencer B, Kosberg K, Fields JA, Stafa K, Adame A, Lashuel H, Frydman J, Shen K, Masliah E, Gitler AD. Parkinson's disease genes VPS35 and EIF4G1 interact genetically and converge on α-synuclein. Neuron. 2015;**85**(1):76-87

[19] Johnson NR, Condello C, Guan S, Oehler A, Becker J, Gavidia M, Carlson GA, Giles K, Prusiner SB. Evidence for sortilin modulating regional accumulation of human tau prions in transgenic mice. Proceedings of the National Academy of Sciences. 2017;**114**(51):E11029-E11036

[20] Dodson SE, Gearing M, Lippa CF, Montine TJ, Levey AI, Lah JJ. LR11/SorLA expression is reduced in sporadic Alzheimer disease but not in familial Alzheimer disease. Journal of Neuropathology and Experimental Neurology. 2006;**65**(9):866-872

[21] Dodson SE, Andersen OM, Karmali V, Fritz JJ, Cheng D, Peng J, Levey AI, Willnow TE, Lah JJ, Disease N. Loss of LR11/SORLA enhances early pathology in a mouse model of amyloidosis: Evidence for a proximal role in Alzheimer's disease. Journal of Neurobiology. 2009;**28**(48):12877-12886

[22] Andersen OM, Reiche J, Schmidt V, Gotthardt M, Spoelgen R, Behlke J, von Arnim CAF, Breiderhoff T, Jansen P, Wu X, Bales KR, Cappai R, Masters CL, Gliemann J, Mufson EJ, Hyman BT, Paul SM, Nykjaer A, Willnow TE. Neuronal sorting protein-related receptor sorLA/LR11 regulates processing of the amyloid precursor protein. Proceedings of the National Academy of Sciences of the United States of America. 2005;**102**(38):13461-13466

[23] Reitz C, Cheng R, Rogaeva E, Lee JH, Tokuhiro S, Zou F, Bettens K, Sleegers K, Tan EK, Kimura R, Shibata N, Arai H, Kamboh MI, Prince JA, Maier W, Riemenschneider M, Owen M, Harold D, Hollingworth P, Cellini E, Sorbi S, Nacmias B, Takeda M, Pericak-Vance MA, Haines JL, Younkin S, Williams J, van Broeckhoven C, Farrer LA, St George-Hyslop PH, Mayeux R. Meta-analysis of the association between variants in SORL1 and Alzheimer disease. Archives of Neurology. 2011;**68**:1, 99-106

[24] Reitz C, Tosto G, Vardarajan B, Rogaeva E, Ghani M, Rogers RS, Conrad C, Haines JL, Pericak-Vance

MA, Fallin MD, Foroud T, Farrer LA, Schellenberg GD, George-Hyslop PS, Mayeux R. Independent and epistatic effects of variants in VPS10-d receptors on Alzheimer disease risk and processing of the amyloid precursor protein (APP). Translational Psychiatry. 2013;**3**(5):e256-e256

[25] Hermey G. The Vps10p-domain receptor family. Cellular and Molecular Life Sciences. 2009;**66**(16):2677-2689

[26] Sarnataro D, Caputo A, Casanova P, Puri C, Paladino S, Tivodar SS, Campana V, Tacchetti C, Zurzolo C. Lipid rafts and clathrin cooperate in the internalization of PrP in epithelial FRT cells. PLoS One. 2009;**4**(6):e5829

[27] Nielsen MS, Madsen P, Christensen EI, Nykjær A, Gliemann J, Kasper D, Pohlmann R, Petersen CM. The sortilin cytoplasmic tail conveys Golgi-endosome transport and binds the VHS domain of the GGA2 sorting protein. The EMBO Journal. 2001;**20**(9):2180-2190

[28] Bonifacino JTL. Signals for sorting of transmembrane proteins for endosomes and lysosomes. Annual Review of Biochemistry. 2003;**72**:395-447

[29] Sunyach C, Jen A, Deng J, Fitzgerald K, Frobert Y, Grassi J, Mccaffrey M, Morris R. The mechanism of internalisation of glycosylphosphatidylinositol-anchored prion protein. The EMBO Journal. 2003;**22**(14):3591-3601

[30] Ren K, Gao C, Zhang J, Wang K, Xu Y, Bin Wang S, Wang H, Tian C, Shi Q, Dong XP. Flotillin-1 mediates PrPC endocytosis in the cultured cells during Cu^{2+} stimulation through molecular interaction. Molecular Neurobiology. 2013;**48**(3):631-646

Chapter 4

Prion Protein Strain Diversity and Disease Pathology

Saima Zafar, Neelam Younas, Mohsin Shafiq and Inga Zerr

Abstract

The infectious agents, prions, are composed mainly of conformational isomers of the cellular prion protein (PrPc) in its abnormal accumulated scrapie forms (PrPSc). The distinct prion isolates or strains have been associated with different PrPSc prion protein conformations and patterns of glycosylation and are associated with disease progression and severity. In humans, sporadic Creutzfeldt-Jakob disease (sCJD) is the most common form and has been divided into six subtypes, based on PrPSc electrophoretic mobility and allelic variation at codon 129, among which sCJD MM1 and sCJD VV2 are the two most commonly occurring subtypes with known clinical manifestations. The strain-specific response of PrPSc suggests both the molecular classification and the pathogenesis of prion diseases along with posttranslational modification of PrP in humans and animals.

Keywords: prion strain, CJD, conformation, dynamics, aggregation

1. Introduction

For the last two decades, scientists have been working on the prion-related diseases, though major features of this transmissible neurodegenerative disease are still not clear. Among some ambiguities, the prion strain phenomenon and the zoonotic potential are the most discussed and enigmatic questions.

Prion diseases are fatal neurodegenerative disorder linked with misfolding of the host-derived protein, named prion protein. The prevalence of the disease in human population is very low (i.e., ~1–2 cases per million) and affect typically aged people. Among this 15% showed genetic concomitant, i.e., point mutation in *PRNP* gene.

Prion diseases are also well-known risk factor for ruminants, including sheep and goats with scrapie, cattle with bovine spongiform encephalopathy, and recently cervids with chronic wasting diseases (CWD). The prion agent was not able to cross the species barriers between humans and ruminant to a high extent, until the new application livestock carcasses recycling into the ruminant alimentary chain. This new implementation resulted in partial inactivation of the BSE prions and cemented the approach with zoonotic potential and spread in humans. This outbreak was famous as the mad cow disease in cattle and the variant CJD (vCJD) in humans. The prion strain diversity, potential to adapt from one host to another, is a mysterious character-impelled scientific community to uncover the concealed story behind.

2. General background

2.1 The prion protein

Cellular form of prion protein PrPc (prion protein) also referred to as CD 230 (cluster of differentiation 230) is coded from *PRNP* gene on the short arm of chromosome 20. The *PRNP* gene of mammals contains three exons. The open reading frame (ORF) lies entirely within exon 3 which transcribes mRNA (2.1–2.5 kb length) with approximately 50 copies/cell in neurons [1, 2]. Physiological involvement of prion protein is diverse, but the active contribution is reflected by the high level of *PRNP* sequence similarity and conservation across the species in mammals. The expression of PrPc is ubiquitous in mammals' bodies, with the highest levels in immune regulatory cells and masses, suggesting a high degree of metabolic involvement in both systems [3].

Cellular prion protein exists in multiple conformations in the cell. In humans, the newly synthesized and unprocessed PrPc is approximately 253 amino acids in length and has a molecular weight of 35–36 kDa. Mature PrPc, after posttranslational modifications, the physiological form of PrP constitutes 208 amino acid residues. PrPc is translocated to the ER lumen due to the presence of N-terminal signal peptide. Glycophosphotidyl (GPI) anchor is added after the removal of C-terminal signal peptide. After the addition of GPI anchor, PrPc is associated to the lipid rafts. Raft association of PrPc is necessary for the proper folding and glycosylation (at two asparagine residues, i.e., Asn 181 and Asn 197) taking place in ER [4] and formation of a disulfide linkage between the two cysteine residues, i.e., 179 and 214, in human PrP in the Golgi apparatus [5]. In addition, mature PrPc contains five octapeptide repeats with a sequence PHGGGWGQ near NH_2-terminal that are encoded by codons 51–91 of the *PRNP* gene [6]. Physiological form of prion protein, PrPc, occurs predominantly along with the truncated, transmembrane COOH–terminal and transmembrane NH_2-terminal forms, namely, PrP^{Ctm} and PrP^{Ntm}, respectively, due to transmembrane insertion of the hydrophobic pocket between aa 110 and 134 [7, 8]. A GPI anchor is attached to PrPc during its life cycle in the cell [9].

In neurons, the cell surface retentivity is very short-lived, like other classical membrane receptors, i.e., a $t_{1/2}$ of 3–5 min. The endocytosis is rather enigmatic. In different cells and different physiological conditions, internalization via both clathrin- and non-clathrin-coated vesicles is reported [10].

Structural studies of recombinant human PrPc reveal that the protein consists of three α-helices at aa residues 144–154, 175–193, and 200–219 and two small antiparallel β-sheets between aa residues 128–131 and 161–164 [11]. PrPc contains a flexible domain at N-terminal between amino acid positions 23–120, whereas a folded domain at C-terminal between amino acids 121–231.

The presence of the PrPc on cell surface suggests its role as a cell receptor. Many studies relate PrPc to diverse signaling pathways. The N-terminal domain containing the octapeptide repetitive motif is reported to exhibit a high affinity for copper ions (Cu^{2+}), suggesting the involvement of PrPc in copper metabolism [12, 13]. PrP is also reported to regulate the influx of Zn^{2+} into the neuronal cells via α-amino-3-hydroxy-5-methyl-4-isoxazolepropionate (AMPA) receptors, by acting as a zinc sensor to the AMPA receptor acting as transporter for Zn^{2+}. These results also suggest that PrP-mediated zinc uptake may contribute to neurodegeneration in prion and other neurodegenerative diseases [14, 15]. PrPc also promotes cellular Ca^{2+} influx via VGCC [16, 17]. Likewise, the activation of Ras GTPases after interaction of PrPc leading to Erk activation is also reported [18]. Activation of protein kinase C and PI3 kinase/Akt signaling is also reported to be associated to PrP, but the mechanism of activation is poorly understood [19, 20].

Derivatives resulting from the various PrPc-proteolytic cleavages are associated to the alteration of PrPc physiology. An α-cleavage at aa residues 110/111 results in N1 and C1 fragments, whereas a β-cleavage event at aa residue 90 results in N2 and C2 fragments. On the cell surface, some proportion of PrPc also undergoes an ADAM10-driven cleavage at GPI anchor called as shedding, resulting in the release of full-length PrPc molecule in extracellular milieu [21].

2.2 Prion diseases

Prion diseases, also known as transmissible spongiform encephalopathies (TSEs), are rare progressive, incurable fatal neurodegenerative diseases that have the property of transmissibility [2, 22, 23]. Prion diseases affect humans and animals. Human prion diseases include Creutzfeldt-Jakob disease (CJD), fatal familial insomnia (FFI), Gerstmann-Sträussler-Scheinker syndrome, variably protease-sensitive prionopathy (VPSPr), vCJD, and Iatrogenic CJD (iCJD) [24]. Animal prion diseases include bovine spongiform encephalopathy (BSE) in cattle [25], chronic wasting disease (CWD) in deer and elk [26], and scrapie in sheep, goats and experimentally infected rodents [12].

Human prion diseases occur at a rate of one to two cases per million per year. Among human prion diseases, 80–95% are sporadic Creutzfeldt-Jakob disease (sCJD), 10–15% are genetic (often familial), and less than 1% are acquired. In sCJD, the conversion of PrPc to PrPSc is thought to occur spontaneously (or possibly through a somatic mutation of *PRNP*). In genetic prion diseases, it is thought that mutations in the prion protein gene, *PRNP*, make the PrPc more susceptible to changing conformation (misfolding) into PrPSc. In acquired forms, PrPSc is accidentally transmitted to a person, causing their endogenous PrPc to misfold [27].

Prion diseases belong to a growing family of protein misfolding diseases that are attributed to misfolding (conformational alterations) and aggregation of proteins in specific brain regions, including Alzheimer's disease, Parkinson's disease, and systemic amyloidosis [28, 29]. Some characteristic features of prion diseases are their wide phenotypic heterogeneity and their multiple modes of occurrence (sporadic, genetic, or acquired) [30, 31]. Central hypothesis in prion diseases is the conversion of an endogenous protease-sensitive cellular prion protein, PrPc, into a conformationally altered self-replicating protease-resistant pathological isoform, PrPSc [32], in the central and lymphoreticular systems. PrPSc binds to cellular PrPc and catalyzes its conversion to an infectious form by nucleation and fragmentation cycle [33]. Prions are resistant to proteases, heat, and decontamination treatments, which is a major challenge for the prevention of prion diseases. Although protease-resistant prions correlate only slightly with infectivity, infectivity is linked to protease-sensitive oligomers [34]. PrPc-to-PrPSc conversion brings in neurotoxicity to the attributes of PrPSc [35]. Diseases arising due to prion misfolding are enlisted in **Table 1**.

Human prion diseases are characterized by a range of clinical symptoms and are classified by both clinico-pathological symptoms and etiology, with subclassifications according to the molecular features. Clinical manifestations include spongiform degeneration, motor and cognitive impairments, neuronal loss, gliosis, astrocytosis, and neuronal dysfunction [23]. Prion diseases have long incubation periods; once clinical symptoms appear, disease progresses very rapidly with lethality in all cases.

Sporadic Creutzfeldt-Jakob disease (sCJD) has average survival of about 6 months, with 85–90% of patients dying within 1 year. The peak age of onset is 55–75 years of age, with median age of onset of about 67 years and mean of 64 years [36]. Sporadic Creutzfeldt-Jakob disease has been classified based on combination of two features: a *PRNP* polymorphism at codon M129V [37] and the size of PK-digested PrPSc on Western blot giving two main types: type 1, with a more distal

	Phenotypes
Familial (inherited)	Familial Creutzfeldt-Jakob-disease (fCJD)
	Fatal familial insomnia (FFI)
	Gerstmann-Sträussler-Scheinker disease (GSS)
	Mixed or undefined forms
Sporadic	CJD (sporadic)
	Typical (MM1 and MV1)
	Early onset (VV1)
	Long duration (MM2)
	Kuru plaques (MV2)
	Ataxic (VV2)
	Sporadic familial insomnia (sFI)
Acquired	Kuru
	Iatrogenic CJD (iCJD)
	variant CJD (vCJD)
Modified [93].	

Table 1.
Classification of human prion disease.

cleavage site, are 21 kDa and type 2, with a more proximal cleavage site, are 19 kDa. These factors result in six possible combinations (MM1, MV1, VV1, MM2, MV2, and VV2) [36]. Codon 129 M/M homozygosity is reported to be associated with an early-onset and aggressive dementia in the CJD patients, whereas V/V homozygosity correlates to a more prolonged pathology with ataxic onset [38]. Apart from codon 129, two other polymorphisms have been reported, i.e., N171S and E219K [39, 40]. Disease-specific PrP mutations have been reviewed in detail by [41]. GSS associated *PRNP* mutations include P102L, P105L, A117V, F198S, D202N, Q212P, and Q217R. *PRNP* mutations associated to fCJD include P102L, P105L, A117V, F198S, D202N, Q212P, and Q217R, whereas a single missense mutation (D178N) has been reported for FFI. This vast structural diversity and switching to disease causing PrPSc make prion protein and its derivatives interesting subject of study.

Although many laboratories are working on therapeutic strategies for prion disease, still they are incurable although some of the symptoms can be temporarily treated [27]. Three randomized double-blinded placebo-controlled trials have failed to alter disease outcome [27, 42].

3. Prion strains and impact on biological parameters

3.1 Prion strain diversity

Prion diseases affect a range of mammalian species and are caused by misfolding of normal cellular PrPc to self-propagating pathological isoform (PrPSc) [43]. Prions can form several distinct self-templating conformers, called prion strains (or variants), which confer dramatic variation in disease pathology and transmission [44]. Diverse strains of prions [45] exist and are operationally defined by differences in a heritable phenotype under controlled experimental transmission setups. Prion strains can differ in tissue tropism, incubation period, clinical signs of disease, and host range.

Prion disorders remain a challenge to modern science in the twenty-first century because of their strain diversity and interspecies transmission properties. Different clinicopathological properties of prion ailments are associated to biochemical heterogeneity in pathogenic protein. Unfortunately, little is known about the mechanisms that drive these differences in biochemical properties.

The mechanism by which a protein pathogen can encode strain diversity is only beginning to be understood. The identification of strain-specific cellular cofactors persuading the generation of new prion strains or the selection, from a conformationally heterogeneous population of PrPSc, of the most suitable prion conformation in a specific environment, denotes an important milestone toward the understanding of the mechanisms of prion strain diversity, which can have vital clinical and therapeutic implications. Adaptation to a new host is the basis of interspecies transmission of prion infections. In some cases, no abnormally folded PrP is found, reflecting a molecular species barrier to disease transmission [46, 47].

Although significant advancements have been made in comprehending the phenomenon of prion strains, many pieces of information are still missing, most important among them is the definitive evidence for the structural differences between prion strains and the relationship between the strain-specific properties of PrPSc and the resulting phenotype of disease [48, 49].

There are two main theories about possible interspecies transmission and adaptive properties of prion infections: the first one considers that strains are present as a single clone in inoculum, and if a new strain arises, it can be assumed that a stain shift has occurred. The second one considers that strains exist as a pool of different molecular species with a dominant type of PrPSc that is preferentially propagated in a given host, but in a different host, a minor PrPSc type can be favored, causing a shift in the strain. The second theory seems to better explain the high level of strain diversity that is reported from experimental data, although the likelihood that prion strains can infect the host as a single clone cannot be excluded. Plausible explanation for the second theory can be that from a pool of different conformations of PrPSc, only a specific fraction is able to replicate in a certain host species, in a manner that is dependent on the sequence and conformation of the PrPc, on the natural clearance capacity of the infected cells [50–53] and on the presence of cofactors [54–56]. In such a model, a prion strain behaves as a quasi-species and represents a pool of molecules that are kept under control by the host [57]. Hence, in a given host, a strain will be constituted of a principal molecular component and a minor one.

Accordingly, interspecies transmission depends on compatibility between the conformation of pathological PrPSc and of the PrPc of the new host, on cell and tissue environment and cofactors [58, 59]. When a prion strain of one species infects an animal of a different species, there are two possible outcomes. The first is that the pathological PrPSc has no conformation compatibility with the host PrPc, resulting in non-conversion; in this case, the species barrier is defined as absolute. The second possibility is that the PrPSc conformation is compatible with the PrPc host conformation, allowing conversion and, ultimately, infection. In this case the proliferated strain can be identical to the infecting unit [60] or can change into a conformationally different strain due to cellular environment, polymorphisms, and cofactors [58, 59]. So, this type of transmission can facilitate the replication of the minor molecular component, if it is favored in the new host, or the generation of a new PrPSc different from the one of the inoculum [61, 62].

Many studies have been performed to reveal the nature of the cofactors that may be involved. It has been demonstrated that RNA molecules; protein chaperones, such as Hsp104 and GroEL; and others have been shown to change strain properties of prions highlighting the role of different cofactors in determining prion strain' propagation properties.

3.2 Transmissibility, heritable phenotype, and species barrier

In the early 1900s, the intraspecies transmission of the TSE agent was first documented with sheep scrapie [63]. The intraspecies transmission (i.e., sheep-sheep) showed marked attack rate as compared to the cross species transmission (i.e., sheep-mice) which showed incomplete attack rate and longer incubation periods. In cross species transmissions, the main hindrance was the adaptation of prion to its new host that leads to the vitiated prions after few subpassages, i.e., 2–3 passages. Previously, this phenomenon hindered the development of rodent models. Later, it has been reported that distinct prion strains, upon serial adaptation of sheep or goat scrapie isolates, could be raised and propagate in different lines of mice. The incubation time, disease severity, and vacuolation distribution in the brain of the mice-adapted strains showed marked signature of the specific disease [64]. However, the major goal at that time was to establish disease-specific end-stage response with clinical symptomatic phase leading to the anatomic distribution with significant lesion score profile. The first experiments reported inoculation of sheep scrapie to goats [65–67]. By that time, prion transmission from one species to the other, i.e., mink to small ruminants, was reported [68], and the bank vole showed maximum transmission capability and turned out as the universal prion strain acceptor [69–71]. In contrast, few studies also reported partial species barriers to pass prions from one species to another, i.e., scrapie isolates to cattle [72].

The emerging field of engineered transgenic mouse models, in combination with endogenous mouse PrP expression (presence or absence), significantly enhanced the possibilities for studying the zoonotic potential of prions [73–76]. In many cases, these experimental setups made emerged the idea that almost every prion could adapt to almost every PrP substrate, provided that some critical parameters have been set up in order to adapt the strain to its new host PrP [77–79]. The transmission efficacy of vCJD strain to wild-type mice also showed conserved and uniform characteristic BSE strain phenotype. The incubation period, glycoform analysis, and lesion profile did not show differential alterations in brain regions and in lymphoreticular tissue [80].

4. Prion strains and disease response

4.1 Phenotypic variants of PrP and human prion strains

The cellular prion protein is a product of *PRNP* gene-residing the chromosome 20 in human. The conformational variations of PrPc in transmissible spongiform encephalopathies (TSEs) give rise to multiple phenotypic variants of PrP-scrapie form (PrPSc), referred to as prion strains. A pure strain refers to a molecular population of PrPSc with characteristic features such as incubation time, PrPSc distribution patterns, resultant spongiosis, and relative severity of the spongiform changes in the brain, when inoculated into distinct host species. In a given prion pathology, a strain species predominantly exists along with minimal concentrations of strains. Classically prion strains are classified based on abovementioned features. Characteristic pattern of prion strains on the western blotting has also been used for the strain classification. The differences of western blotting patterns occur due to the variability of proteinase k cleavage sites in prion protein and abundance of differential PrP glycoforms (i.e., di-glycosylated, mono-glycosylated, and unglycosylated isoforms). Rather recently, nontrivial approaches such as seeding potential of prion variants and differential strain-specific oligomeric populations have expanded the spectrum of strain classification [81].

In human prion strains, variation is determined by proteinase K (PK) resistance. PK-resistant PrP occurs in two forms based on the migration on western blots, i.e., PrPSc type 1 migrates at 21 kDa, whereas type 2 PrPSc migrates at 19 kDa (resultant of two distinct PK digestion at amino acids 96 and 85, respectively) [82]. Atypical cases of variably protease-sensitive prionopathy (VPSPr) exhibit a different sensitivity profile to the Proteinase K. Some cases have been reported to exhibit no PK resistance (viz., protease-sensitive prionopathy, PSPr), whereas some other VPSPr cases present less PK resistance resulting in a ladder-like pattern on western blot ranging from 27 to 7 kDa. Details of human prion strains in combination with codon 129 M/V polymorphism are listed in **Table 2** [83].

4.2 Templating activity

Prion templating activity coupled with the structure studies is also used as an index for strain classification. Baskakov and colleagues have been able to differentiate the hamster recombinant PrP strains based on the structure profiles formed under different conditions, i.e., R and S fibrils, result of polymerization while rotating and shaking the monomers, respectively [84]. Structural validations of the prion protein polymers are challenging due to overly high hydrophobic nature of the polymers. For robust templating activity-based classification of prion strains, two methods have been established, namely, protein misfolding cyclic amplification (PMCA) and real-time quacking-induced cyclic amplification (RT-QuIC), where prion strains are utilized as templates for the recombinant prion protein. Templating in PMCA is usually validated with downstream Western blotting, where RT-QuIC is a fluorometry-based method and provides the real-time information, utilizing thioflavin-T binding to polymers. Lag phase and final fluorescence signals could be used for discrimination between different prion strains [71]. RT-QuIC

Strain type	Histological characteristics	Disease subtype, % age occurrence of all prion pathologies
MM/MV 1	Diffuse synaptic deposits	sCJD, 40%
VV 2	Perineuronal and cerebellar plaque-like deposits	sCJD, 15%
MV 2K	Kuru plaques	sCJD, 8%
MM 2C	Cortical confluent vacuoles	sCJD, 1%
MM 2T (sFI)	Thalamo-olivary atrophy	sCJD
VV 1	Corticostriatal synaptic deposits	sCJD
MM 2V (vCJD)	Florid plaques	sCJD
MM/MV1+2C	Mixed diffuse synaptic deposits and cortical confluent vacuoles	sCJD, 30%
MV 2K+C	Mixed Kuru plaques and cortical confluent vacuoles	sCJD
MM-VPSPr	Large vacuoles, PrPSc microplaques in the molecular layer of the cerebellum, as well as target-like rounded formations of clusters of granules that increase in size toward the center	VPSPr
MV-VPSPr		
VV-VPSPr		

Modified from [83].
Abbreviations: BSE, bovine spongiform encephalopathy; sCJD, sporadic Creutzfeldt-Jakob disease; sFI, sporadic fatal insomnia; VPSPr, variably protease-sensitive prionopathy; gCJD, genetic CJD; GSS, Gerstmann-Sträussler-Scheinker disease; FFI, fatal familial insomnia; vCJD, variant CJD.

Table 2.
Human prion strain histopathological profiles, influenced by codon 129 polymorphism determined in different backgrounds of human transmissible spongiform encephalopathies (TSEs).

proves to be a highly specific and sensitive method and has been utilized to establish strain differences of typical and atypical prionopathies, e.g., the L-type BSE and classical BSEs [85].

A recent report showed oligo-/poly-thiophene derivate as a potent fluorescent approach to discriminate between prion strains [86]. The excitation/emission spectra were obtained from the CWD and scrapie strains, and the interactive association between thiophene and different aggregates were used in combination with conformational restriction to characterize different strains.

4.3 Distribution of density variants

Prion strain polymerization is a sequential process where single molecules are converted to polymers via a multitude of conformational variants. Different prion strains have been identified in animal and human cases based upon differential population densities of these quaternary structures [87]. Quaternary structure conformers of PrP have been isolated and studied using sucrose density gradient by many groups [88–91]. Differential prion strains have been also identified for the rapidly progressive forms of Alzheimer's disease with distinct population of high-density PrP oligomeric species [92].

5. Conclusions and future outlook

Prion strains and the interspecies barriers are still enigmatic phenomena. One of the surprising things about prion protein is that this single protein can fold up in

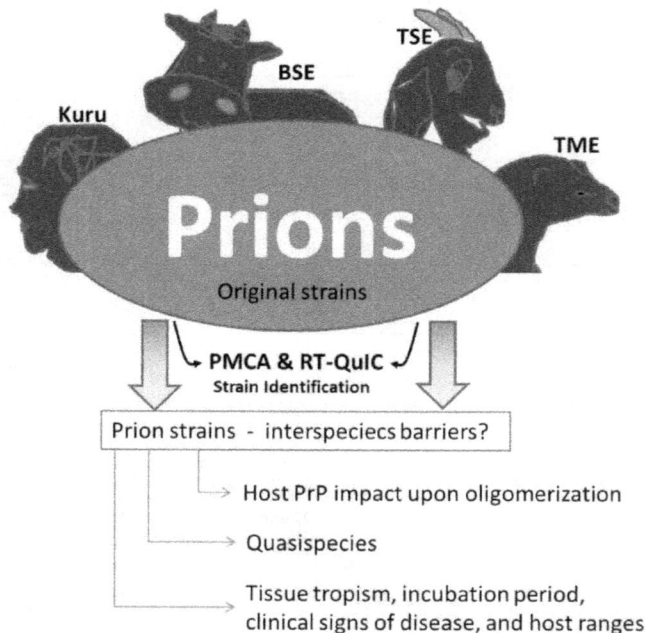

Figure 1.
Prion strain emergence and interspecies transmission. The original prion strains were named as Kuru in human, BSE in cows, TSE in goat and sheep, and TME in minks. PMCA and RT-QuiC mobilized the prion strain characterization. The interspecies transmission of prions linked with host PrP oligomerization role, appearance of subassemblies named as quasispecies, tissue tropism, incubation period of prions, symptomatic stages of the diseases, and host range.

so many different ways that are toxic and cause disease. Recent advances in PrPSc amplification methods, i.e., PMCA and RT-QuIC, might lead to clear improvements in the characterization of the prion strain.

From last many years, prion protein strain characterization and impact on disease are under debate. The use of prion transgenic models has been influential for studying and clarifying the molecular mechanisms in which the protein is involved. The ability to cross species barrier may be a result of either quasispecies theory or host PrP impact on progressive templating deformation upon oligomerization theory (**Figure 1**). These phenomena are mostly time dependent. By learning the structural variation and potential interspecies transmissions, we may progress toward the understanding of disease pathology and subsequently development of novel therapeutic approaches to such devastating disorders.

Acknowledgements

The study was performed within the recently established Clinical Dementia Center at the University Medical Hospital Goettingen and was partly supported by grants from the EU Joint Program Neurodegenerative Disease Research (JPND ± DEMTEST) (Biomarker-based diagnosis of rapid progressive dementias-optimization of diagnostic protocols, 01ED1201A). This work was supported by a grant from Helmholtz-Alberta Initiative-Infectious Diseases Research (HAI-IDR) and APRI-Human prions distinguishing sporadic from familial forms via structure and function as well as from the DZNE clinical project (Helmholtz).

Conflict of interest

We have no conflict of interest to declare.

Author details

Saima Zafar[1,2]*, Neelam Younas[1,2], Mohsin Shafiq[1,2] and Inga Zerr[1,2]*

1 Department of Neurology, Clinical Dementia Center, University Medical Center Goettingen (UMG), Georg-August University, Goettingen, Germany

2 German Center for Neurodegenerative Diseases (DZNE), Goettingen, Germany

*Address all correspondence to: sz_awaan@yahoo.com
and ingazerr@med.uni-goettingen.de

IntechOpen

References

[1] Liao YC, Lebo RV, Clawson GA, Smuckler EA. Human prion protein cDNA: Molecular cloning, chromosomal mapping, and biological implications. Science (80-). 1986;**233**:364-367

[2] Prusiner SB. Molecular biology of prion diseases. Science (80). 1991;**252**:1515-1522. DOI: 10.1126/science.1675487

[3] Linden R, Martins VR, Prado MAM, Cammarota M, Izquierdo I, Brentani RR. Physiology of the prion protein. Physiological Reviews. 2008;**88**:673-728. DOI: 10.1152/physrev.00007.2007

[4] Haraguchi T, Fisher S, Olofsson S, Endo T, Groth D, Tarentino A, et al. Asparagine-linked glycosylation of the scrapie and cellular prion proteins. Archives of Biochemistry and Biophysics. 1989;**274**:1-13. DOI: 10.1016/0003-9861(89)90409-8

[5] Turk E, Teplow DB, Hood LE, Prusiner SB. Purification and properties of the cellular and scrapie hamster prion proteins. European Journal of Biochemistry. 1988;**176**:21-30. DOI: 10.1111/j.1432-1033.1988.tb14246.x

[6] Owen F, Poulter M, Shah T, Collinge J, Lofthouse R, Baker H, et al. An in-frame insertion in the prion protein gene in familial Creutzfeldt-Jakob disease. Brain Research. Molecular Brain Research. 1990;7:273-276

[7] Hegde RS. A transmembrane form of the prion protein in neurodegenerative disease. Science (80-). 1998;**279**:827-834. DOI: 10.1126/science.279.5352.827

[8] Hegde RS, Voigt S, Lingappa VR. Regulation of protein topology by trans-acting factors at the endoplasmic reticulum. Molecular Cell. 1998;2:85-91. DOI: 10.1016/S1097-2765(00)80116-1

[9] Taylor DR, Hooper NM. The prion protein and lipid rafts. Molecular Membrane Biology. 2006;**23**:89-99. DOI: 10.1080/09687860500449994

[10] Sunyach C. The mechanism of internalization of glycosylphosphatidylinositol-anchored prion protein. The EMBO Journal. 2003;**22**:3591-3601. DOI: 10.1093/emboj/cdg344

[11] Surewicz WK, Apostol MI. Prion protein and its conformational conversion: A structural perspective. Topics in Current Chemistry. 2011;**305**:135-168. DOI: 10.1007/128_2011_165

[12] Stockel J, Safar J, Wallace AC, Cohen FE, Prusiner SB. Prion protein selectively binds copper (II) ions. Biochemistry. 1998;**37**:7185-7193. DOI: 10.1021/bi972827k

[13] Dobson CM. Structural biology: Prying into prions. Nature. 2005;**345**:747-749. DOI: 10.1038/435747a

[14] He Q, Meiri KF. Isolation and characterization of detergent-resistant microdomains responsive to NCAM-mediated signaling from growth cones. Molecular and Cellular Neurosciences. 2002;**19**:18-31. DOI: 10.1006/mcne.2001.1060

[15] Cooper DMF, Crossthwaite AJ. Higher-order organization and regulation of adenylyl cyclases. Trends in Pharmacological Sciences. 2006;**27**:426-431. DOI: 10.1016/j.tips.2006.06.002

[16] Herms JW, Korte S, Gall S, Schneider I, Dunker S, Kretzschmar HA. Altered intracellular calcium homeostasis in cerebellar granule cells of prion protein-deficient mice. Journal of Neurochemistry. 2000;**75**:1487-1492. DOI: 10.1046/j.1471-4159.2000.0751487

[17] Fuhrmann M, Bittner T, Mitteregger G, Haider N, Moosmang S, Kretzschmar H, et al. Loss of the cellular prion protein affects the Ca2+ homeostasis in hippocampal CA1 neurons. Journal of Neurochemistry. 2006;**98**:1876-1885

[18] Stork PJS, Schmitt JM. Crosstalk between cAMP and MAP kinase signaling in the regulation of cell proliferation. Trends in Cell Biology. 2002;**12**:258-266. DOI: 10.1016/S0962-8924(02)02294-8

[19] Dekker LV, Palmer RH, Parker PJ. The protein kinase C and protein kinase C related gene families. Current Opinion in Structural Biology. 1995;**5**:396-402. Available from: http://www.ncbi.nlm.nih.gov/pubmed/7583639

[20] Vassallo N, Herms J, Behrens C, Krebs B, Saeki K, Onodera T, et al. Activation of phosphatidylinositol 3-kinase by cellular prion protein and its role in cell survival. Biochemical and Biophysical Research Communications. 2005;**332**:75-82. DOI: 10.1016/j.bbrc.2005.04.099

[21] Altmeppen HC, Puig B, Dohler F, Thurm DK, Falker C, Krasemann S. Proteolytic processing of the prion protein in health and disease. American Journal of Neurodegenerative Disease. 2012;**1**:15-31

[22] Caughey B, Chesebro B. Transmissible spongiform encephalopathies and prion protein interconversions. Advances in Virus Research. 2001;**56**:277-311

[23] Collinge J. Prion diseases of humans and animals: Their causes and molecular basis. Annual Review of Neuroscience. 2001;**24**:519-550

[24] Aguzzi A, Calella AM. Prions: Protein aggregation and infectious diseases. Physiological Reviews. 2009;**89**:1105-1152. DOI: 10.1152/physrev.00006.2009

[25] Hope J, Reekie LJ, Hunter N, Multhaup G, Beyreuther K, White H, et al. Fibrils from brains of cows with new cattle disease contain scrapie-associated protein. Nature. 1988;**336**:390-392. DOI: 10.1038/336390a0

[26] Williams ES, Young S. Chronic wasting disease of captive mule deer: A spongiform encephalopathy. Journal of Wildlife Diseases. 1980;**16**:89-98

[27] Brown K, Mastrianni JA. The prion diseases. Journal of Geriatric Psychiatry and Neurology. 2010;**23**(4):277-298. DOI: 10.1177/0891988710383576

[28] Soto C. Unfolding the role of protein misfolding in neurodegenerative diseases. Nature Reviews. Neuroscience. 2003;**4**:49-60. DOI: 10.1038/nrn1007

[29] Aguzzi A, Rajendran L. The transcellular spread of cytosolic amyloids, prions, and prionoids. Neuron. 2009;**64**:783-790. DOI: 10.1016/j.neuron.2009.12.016

[30] McKintosh E, Tabrizi SJ, Collinge J. Prion diseases. Journal of Neurovirology. 2003;**9**:183-193

[31] Prusiner SB. Novel proteinaceous infectious particles cause scrapie. Science. 1982;**216**:136-144

[32] Caughey B. Prion protein conversions: Insight into mechanisms, TSE transmission barriers and strains. British Medical Bulletin. 2003;**66**:109-120

[33] Knowles TPJ et al. An analytical solution to the kinetics of breakable filament assembly. Science. 2009;**326**:1533-1537. DOI: 10.1126/science.1178250

[34] Aguzzi A, Lakkaraju AKK. Cell biology of prions and prionoids: A status report. Trends in Cell Biology. 2016;**26**:40-51. DOI: 10.1016/j.tcb.2015.08.007

[35] Norrby E. Prions and protein-folding diseases. Journal of Internal Medicine. 2011;**270**:1-14. DOI: 10.1111/j.1365-2796.2011.02387

[36] Puoti G, Bizzi A, Forloni G, et al. Sporadic human prion diseases: Molecular insights and diagnosis. Lancet Neurology. 2012;**11**(7):618-628. DOI: 10.1016/S1474-4422(12)70063-7

[37] Lloyd SE, Mead S, Collinge J. Genetics of prion diseases. Current Opinion in Genetics and Development. 2013;**23**:345-351. DOI: 10.1016/j.gde.2013.02.012

[38] Palmer MS, Dryden AJ, Hughes JT, Collinge J. Homozygous prion protein genotype predisposes to sporadic Creutzfeldt-Jakob disease. Nature. 1991;**352**:340-342. DOI: 10.1038/352340a0

[39] Kitamoto T, Tateishi J. Human prion diseases with variant prion protein. Philosophical Transactions of the Royal Society B: Biological Sciences. 1994;**343**:391-398. DOI: 10.1098/rstb.1994.003431

[40] Hizume M, Kobayashi A, Teruya K, Ohashi H, Ironside JW, Mohri S, et al. Human prion protein (PrP) 219K is converted to PrPSc but shows heterozygous inhibition in variant Creutzfeldt-Jakob disease infection. The Journal of Biological Chemistry. 2009;**284**:3603-3609. DOI: 10.1074/jbc.M809254200

[41] Acevedo-Morantes CY, Wille H. The structure of human prions: From biology to structural models—Considerations and pitfalls. Viruses. 2014;**6**:3875-3892. DOI: 10.3390/v6103875

[42] Kim MO, Geschwind MD. Clinical update of Jakob-Creutzfeldt disease. Current Opinion in Neurology. 2015;**28**(3):302-310. DOI: 10.1097/WCO.0000000000000197

[43] Colby DW, Prusiner SB. Prions. Cold Spring Harbor Perspectives in Biology. 2011;**3**(1):a006833. DOI: 10.1101/cshperspect.a006833

[44] Stein KC, True HL. Extensive diversity of prion strains is defined by differential chaperone interactions and distinct amyloidogenic regions. PLoS Genetics. 2014;**10**(5):e1004337. DOI: 10.1371/journal.pgen.1004337

[45] Safar JG. Molecular pathogenesis of sporadic prion diseases in man. Prion. 2012;**6**:108-115. DOI: 10.4161/pri.18666

[46] Katorcha E, Gonzalez-Montalban N, Makarava N, Kovacs GG, Baskakov IV. Prion replication environment defines the fate of prion strain adaptation. PLoS Pathogens. 2018;**14**:e1007093. DOI: 10.1371/journal.ppat.1007093

[47] Igel-Egalon A, Beringue V, Rezaei H, Sibille P. Prion strains and transmission barrier phenomena. Pathogens. 2018;**7**:5. DOI: 10.3390/pathogens7010005

[48] Crowell J, Hughson A, Caughey B, Bessen RA. Host determinants of prion strain diversity independent of prion protein genotype. Journal of Virology. 2015;**89**:10427-10441. DOI: 10.1128/JVI.01586-15

[49] Taguchi Y, Lu L, Marrero-Winkens C, Otaki H, Nishida N, Schatzl HM. Disulfide-crosslink scanning reveals prion-induced conformational changes and prion strain-specific structures of the pathological prion protein PrP(Sc). Journal of Biological Chemistry. 2018;**293**:12730-12740. DOI: 10.1074/jbc.RA117.001633

[50] Safar JG, DeArmond SJ, Kociuba K, Deering C, Didorenko S, Bouzamondo-Bernstein E, et al. Prion clearance in bigenic mice. The Journal of General Virology. 2005;**86**:2913-2923. DOI: 10.1099/vir.0.80947-0

[51] Paar C, Wurm S, Pfarr W, Sonnleitner A, Wechselberger C. Prion protein resides in membrane microclusters of the immunological synapse during lymphocyte activation. European Journal of Cell Biology. 2007;**86**:253-264. DOI: 10.1016/j.ejcb.2007.03.001

[52] Wong E, Cuervo AM. Integration of clearance mechanisms: The proteasome and autophagy. Cold Spring Harbor Perspectives in Biology. 2010;**2**:a006734. DOI: 10.1101/cshperspect.a006734

[53] Mannini B, Cascella R, Zampagni M, van WaardeVerhagen M, Meehan S, Roodveldt C, et al. Molecular mechanisms used by chaperones to reduce the toxicity of aberrant protein oligomers. Proceedings of the National Academy of Sciences of the United States of America. 2012;**109**:12479-12484. DOI: 10.1073/pnas.1117799109

[54] Cohen FE, Pan KM, Huang Z, Baldwin M, Fletterick RJ, Prusiner SB. Structural clues to prion replication. Science. 1994;**264**:530-531. DOI: 10.1126/science.7909169

[55] Deleault NR, Lucassen RW, Supattapone S. RNA molecules stimulate prion protein conversion. Nature. 2003;**425**:717-720. DOI: 10.1038/nature01979

[56] Deleault NR, Walsh DJ, Piro JR, Wang F, Wang X, Ma J, et al. Cofactor molecules maintain infectious conformation and restrict strain properties in purified prions. Proceedings of the National Academy of Sciences of the United States of America. 2012;**109**:E1938-E1946. DOI: 10.1073/ pnas.1206999109

[57] Weissmann C, Li J, Mahal SP, Browning S. Prions on the move. EMBO Reports. 2011;**12**:1109-1117. DOI: 10.1038/embor.2011.192

[58] Hill AF, Collinge J. Prion strains and species barriers. Contributions to Microbiology. 2004;**11**:33-49. DOI: 10.1159/000077061

[59] Hamir AN, Kehrli ME Jr, Kunkle RA, Greenlee JJ, Nicholson EM, Richt JA, et al. Experimental interspecies transmission studies of the transmissible spongiform encephalopathies to cattle: Comparison to bovine spongiform encephalopathy in cattle. Journal of Veterinary Diagnostic Investigation. 2011;**23**:407-420. DOI: 10.1177/1040638711403404

[60] Collinge J, Clarke AR. A general model of prion strains and their pathogenicity. Science. 2007;**318**:930-936. DOI: 10.1126/science.1138718

[61] Bessen RA, Marsh RF. Identification of two biologically distinct strains of transmissible mink encephalopathy in hamsters. The Journal of General Virology. 1992;**73**:329-334. DOI: 10.1099/0022-1317-73-2-329

[62] Bartz JC, Bessen RA, McKenzie D, Marsh RF, Aiken JM. Adaptation and selection of prion protein strain conformations following interspecies transmission of transmissible mink encephalopathy. Journal of Virology. 2000;**74**:5542-5547. DOI: 10.1128/ JVI.74.12.5542-5547.2000

[63] Cuillé J, Chelle PL. La tremblante dumouton est bien inoculable. Comptes Rendus de l'Académie des Sciences. 1938;**206**:78-79

[64] Houston F, Andreoletti O. The zoonotic potential of animal prion diseases. Handbook of Clinical Neurology. 2018;**153**:447-462. DOI: 10.1016/B978-0-444-63945-5.00025-8

[65] Plummer PJ. Scrapie—A disease of sheep: A review of the literature. Canadian Journal of Comparative Medicine and Veterinary Science. 1946;**10**:49-54

[66] Pattison IH, Gordon WS, Millson GC. Experimental production of

scrapie in goats. Journal of Comparative Pathology and Therapeutics. 1959;**69**:300IN19-312IN20

[67] Pattison IH, Millson GC. Scrapie produced experimentally in goats with special reference to the clinical syndrome. Journal of Comparative Pathology. 1961;**71**:101-109

[68] Hadlow WJ, Race RE, Kennedy RC. Experimental infection of sheep and goats with transmissible mink encephalopathy virus. Canadian Journal of Veterinary Research. 1987;**51**:135-144

[69] Nonno R, Bari MAD, Cardone F, Vaccari G, Fazzi P, Dell'Omo G, et al. Efficient transmission and characterization of Creutzfeldt-Jakob disease strains in Bank voles. PLoS Pathogens. 2006;**2**:e12. DOI: 10.1371/journal.ppat.0020012

[70] Watts JC, Giles K, Patel S, Oehler A, DeArmond SJ, Prusiner SB. Evidence that bank vole PrP is a universal acceptor for prions. PLoS Pathogens. 2014;**10**:e1003990

[71] Orrú CD, Groveman BR, Raymond LD, Hughson AG, Nonno R, Zou W, et al. Bank vole prion protein as an apparently universal substrate for RT-QuIC-based detection and discrimination of prion strains. PLOS Pathogens. 2015;**11**:e1004983. DOI: 10.1371/journal.ppat.1004983

[72] Robinson MM, Hadlow WJ, Knowles DP, Huff TP, Lacy PA, Marsh RF, et al. Experimental infection of cattle with the agents of transmissible mink encephalopathy and scrapie. Journal of Comparative Pathology. 1995;**113**:241-251

[73] Collinge J, Palmer MS, Sidle KC, Hill AF, Gowland I, Meads J, et al. Unaltered susceptibility to BSE in transgenic mice expressing human prion protein. Nature. 1995;**378**:779-783

[74] Büeler H, Aguzzi A, Sailer A, Greiner R-A, Autenried P, Aguet M, et al. Mice devoid of PrP are resistant to scrapie. Cell. 1993;**73**:1339-1347

[75] Telling GC, Scott M, Hsiao KK, Foster D, Yang SL, Torchia M, et al. Transmission of Creutzfeldt-Jakob disease from humans to transgenic mice expressing chimeric human-mouse prion protein. Proceedings of the National Academy of Sciences of the United States of America. 1994;**91**:9936-9940

[76] Brandner S, Isenmann S, Raeber A, Fischer M, Sailer A, Kobayashi Y, et al. Normal host prion protein necessary for scrapie-induced neurotoxicity. Nature. 1996;**379**:339-343

[77] Ghaemmaghami S, Watts JC, Nguyen HO, Hayashi S, DeArmond SJ, Prusiner SB. Conformational transformation and selection of synthetic prion strains. Journal of Molecular Biology. 2011;**413**:527-542. DOI: 10.1016/j.jmb.2011.07.021

[78] Baskakov IV. The many shades of prion strain adaptation. Prion. 2011;**8**:27836

[79] Bian J, Khaychuk V, Angers RC, Fernandez-Borges N, Vidal E, Meyerett-Reid C, et al. Prion replication without host adaptation during interspecies transmissions. Proceedings of the National Academy of Sciences of the United States of America. 2017;**114**:1141-1146. DOI: 10.1073/pnas.1611891114.

[80] Ritchie DL, Boyle A, McConnell I, Head MW, Ironside JW, Bruce ME. Transmissions of variant Creutzfeldt-Jakob disease from brain and lymphoreticular tissue show uniform and conserved bovine spongiform encephalopathy-related phenotypic properties on primary and secondary passage in wild-type mice. Journal of

General Virology. 2009;**90**:3075-3082. DOI: 10.1099/vir.0.013227-0

[81] Aguzzi A, Heikenwalder M, Polymenidou M. Insights into prion strains and neurotoxicity. Nature Reviews. Molecular Cell Biology. 2007;**8**:552-561. DOI: 10.1038/nrm2204

[82] Disease SC, Parchi P, Castellani R, Capellari S, Ghetti B, Young K, et al. Molecular basis of phenotypic variability in sporadic Creutzfeldt-Jakob disease. Annals of Neurology. 1996;**39**: 767-778.

[83] Kretzschmar H, Tatzelt J. Prion disease: A tale of folds and strains. Brain Pathology (Zurich, Switzerland).2013;**23**:321-332. DOI: 10.1111/bpa.12045

[84] Makarava N, Ostapchenko VG, Savtchenko R, Baskakov IV. Conformational switching within individual amyloid fibrils. The Journal of Biological Chemistry. 2009;**284**:14386-14395. DOI: 10.1074/jbc.M900533200

[85] Candelise N, Schmitz M, Da Silva Correia SM, Arora AS, Villar-Piqué A, Zafar S, et al. Applications of the real-time quaking-induced conversion assay in diagnosis, prion strain-typing, drug pre-screening and other amyloidopathies. Expert Review of Molecular Diagnostics. 2017;**17**:897-904. DOI: 10.1080/14737159.2017.1368389

[86] Magnusson K, Simon R, Sjölander D, Sigurdson CJ, Hammarström P, Nilsson KPR. Multimodal fluorescence microscopy of prion strain specific PrP deposits stained by thiophene-based amyloid ligands. Prion. 2014;**8**:319-329

[87] Strains P, Phenomena TB. Prion strains and transmission barrier phenomena. Pathogens. 2018;**7**:5. DOI: 10.3390/pathogens7010005

[88] Kim C, Haldiman T, Surewicz K, Cohen Y, Chen W, Blevins J, et al. Small protease sensitive oligomers of PrP^{Sc} in distinct human prions determine conversion rate of PrP^{C}. PLoS pathogens. 2012;**8**:e1002835. DOI: 10.1371/journal.ppat.1002835

[89] Peden AH, Sarode DP, Mulholland CR, Barria MA, Ritchie DL, Ironside JW, et al. The prion protein protease sensitivity, stability and seeding activity in variably protease sensitive prionopathy brain tissue suggests molecular overlaps with sporadic Creutzfeldt-Jakob disease. Acta Neuropathologica Communications. 2014;**2**:1-17. DOI: 10.1186/s40478-014-0152-4

[90] Cohen ML, Kim C, Haldiman T, Elhag M, Mehndiratta P, Pichet T, et al. Rapidly progressive Alzheimer's disease features distinct structures of amyloid-b. Brain. 2015;**138**:1009-1022. DOI: 10.1093/brain/awv006

[91] Hartmann A, Muth C, Dabrowski O, Krasemann S, Glatzel M. Exosomes and the prion protein: More than one truth. Frontiers in Neuroscience. 2017;**11**:1-7. DOI: 10.3389/fnins.2017.00194

[92] Zafar S, Shafiq M, Younas N, Schmitz M, Ferrer I, Zerr I. Prion protein interactome: Identifying novel targets in slowly and rapidly progressive forms of Alzheimer's disease. Journal of Alzheimer's Disease. 2017;**59**:265-275. DOI: 10.3233/JAD-170237

[93] Gambetti P, Kong Q, Zou W, Parchi P, Chen SG. Sporadic and familial CJD: Classification and characterisation. British Medical Bulletin. 2003;**66**:213-239. DOI: 10.1093/bmb/dg66.213

www.ingramcontent.com/pod-product-compliance
Lightning Source LLC
Chambersburg PA
CBHW081243190326
41458CB00016B/5891